Prepare to Push™

What Your Pelvic Floor & Abdomen
Want You to Know about Pregnancy & Birth

Kim Vopni – The Fitness Doula

ISBN 978-0-9947466-0-3
eBook ISBN 978-0-9947466-1-0

First printing October 2015

Edited by Stephanie Fysh
Book design and layout Chelsey Doyle
eBook edition by Bright Wing Books
Photography by Jenn Di Spirito Photography
Illustrations by Tatiana Tushyna

For more information, please contact:

Kim Vopni of Pelvienne Wellness Inc.
(604) 910-3065
kim@pelviennewellness.com

This book is dedicated to my husband, my mother and my children. Thank you to my mom who talked to me about her body and her challenges and for not keeping silent. Thank you to my husband for encouraging me to buy the EPI-NO and for being my biggest fan. Thank you to my children for making me a mother.

Contents

Acknowledgements

I have been taught and mentored by many and this is by no means an exhaustive list but I wanted to acknowledge those who played a particularly prominent role in my work. I have been fortunate to work with some true pioneers, to be inspired by forward thinkers and to have been guided by some truly remarkable people.

Katy Bowman
katysays.com

Diane Lee
babybellybelt.com/about-diane-lee.php

Dr. Bruce Crawford
pfilates.com

Samantha Montpetit-Huynh
belliesinc.com

Julia Di Paolo
belliesinc.com

Kaisa Tuominen
hypopresives.com

Sue Dumais
familypassages.ca

Julie Tupler
diastasisrehab.com

Liz Koch
coreawareness.com

Julie Wiebe
juliewiebept.com

Introduction

Congratulations—you're pregnant! Let the preparations begin! Pregnancy is such an exciting time, and there is so much to prepare for! Most of your focus now is on things like finding a midwife or doctor, maybe hiring a doula, having a baby shower, designing the nursery... You'll read pregnancy books and blogs, join online communities, and download apps. On Pinterest, you'll create a new board filled with images of baby rooms and the latest must-have products. You'll buy an infant car seat (among many other things!), you'll take a prenatal education class, maybe do some yoga (where you'll think of baby names and what colour the baby room should be while holding each pose)... and the list goes on. Most of the to-do's are focused on the baby. But *what about you?*

Preparing you is important too, and preparing your body for birth and motherhood goes far beyond taking folic acid and rubbing belly butter on your tummy to prevent stretch marks. You need to be thinking of your core—how to get it strong for the remainder of your pregnancy, keep it strong for birth, and restore it for motherhood! Unfortunately, many women enter one of the most physically demanding events of their lives ill prepared and are then faced with issues such as mummy tummy, incontinence, and lingering back pain—issues that for the most part can be avoided or at least minimized—and they are left wondering, "Why didn't anyone tell me about this?"

This book changes that. This book prepares you. This book tells you what you need to know—what to do and what not to do—to get through birth in one piece. It will teach you about diastasis recti, the separation of the abdominal muscles that affects most pregnant women. You will also learn about the pelvic floor and how to keep it functioning optimally. **This book gives you the plan: you just need to put it into action!** By following the tips and doing the easy exercises, you will have a more comfortable pregnancy, be empowered for birth, and transition to motherhood with confidence in a body that you love!

CHAPTER ONE

Your Core: Its Parts, Its Roles, Its Ideal Function

Birth is normal and natural—women have been doing it for centuries. But giving birth is like running a marathon, and you wouldn't run a marathon without preparing for it, would you? While birth is natural and your body was designed for it, it can leave your body in an injured state. Unfortunately, because birth is 'natural', often times not enough emphasis is placed on preparing and recovering from birth. Also, we live in an unnatural world where your body has been accustomed to a lifestyle that involves a lot of sitting, and this means that it has developed some compensations that can interfere with the natural birthing process. Hence the need to prepare! Birth is a very physical event: it requires physical and mental stamina. Unfortunately, many women do not train for this big event, leaving them with discomfort in their pregnancies, prolonged and more difficult labours, and an after-baby body that leaves them feeling broken.

Fortunately, with the right information and awareness, you can minimize or eliminate these aches and pains, birth the way you want with more ease and less discomfort, and be confident in your after-baby body. By preparing to push, you are supporting your amazing body as it nurtures and grows your beautiful baby, and you are setting yourself up for a return to optimal function postpartum.

The missing link in childbirth education is the mother's physical preparation for birth, as well as best practices for postpartum healing. Many pregnancy books give you valuable information about what is happening week by week, to both you and your baby, but a lot of critical pieces of information are left out, information that can have a big impact on your pregnancy, your birth experience, and your transition into motherhood. This critical information relates to your inner core—that is, your pelvic floor (actually, your pelvis in general) and your abdomen: the core's two major players.

Your core is the most affected part of your body in pregnancy, during birth, and postpartum, yet it gets little or no attention. Generally, the only thing you may have heard with regards to the pelvic floor is to do your kegels—that's it! No instruction on *how* to do them, no assessment to determine if kegels would even be right for you, no discussion of posture or breathing or alignment and how these affect your ability to do a kegel... just "*Make sure you are doing your kegels.*" You deserve better than that. **Prevention is key, but many women find out only after the fact about core dysfunction and often think it's normal to suffer from things like incontinence and mummy tummy after having kids.** The truth is, many of the challenges new (and seasoned) moms face can be prevented or minimized with the right education and awareness about how to prepare and recover.

As I said earlier, giving birth is like running a marathon, but most women do not prepare for it. Preparation for a physical event such as a marathon involves strength training, stretching and release work, visualization and breathwork. Birth should be no different. The mindset of most is "Millions have done it before me—

it can't be that bad. I'll just hope for the best." Yet once the baby is born, the thinking becomes "I wish I had known that" or "I wish I had paid more attention to my core." By adopting the guidelines in this book, you will follow a different path and make the choice to prepare for your marathon. Good for you!

Learning how to prepare your body for the marathon of birth will set you up for a more comfortable pregnancy and a better birth, and will optimize your return to proper core function postpartum. The basis of the program takes into consideration the principle of specificity, which states that you should train for an event using activities that most closely mimic that event. Now, we can't exactly practise giving birth, but we *can* practise the birth positions, breathing, and visualization, and we can do exercises that support those aspects of birth. This book's program involves getting you connected to your core so that you can train it for pregnancy, so that you can work with it, not against it, in birth, and so that you can then *re*train it once your baby is born. First, though, you need to understand what the true core is. Let's take a look at the core in more detail so you can dive into learning how to best prepare it!

Your Core

The core is made up of a number of muscles that work together to support the spine and pelvis. For our purposes, we will look at the inner core, or what I like to call the *Core 4*.

The Core 4 is made up of, you guessed it, four key players: the breathing diaphragm, the transversus abdominis, the multifidus, and the pelvic floor. This team is designed to work synergistically in anticipation of your every move. That's right—they anticipate and prepare you for the task at hand before you even move! The function of the core is directly tied to the breath, and the breath is directly tied to posture and alignment. If your alignment is off or you are standing or sitting with poor posture, then your breath is not optimized—and, therefore, the function of your core is hindered. Think about a car: if its wheel alignment is off, then the car is less efficient—it burns more gas and the tires wear unevenly. The same thing happens with your body. If your skeletal alignment is not ideal, your body will not work as efficiently, and wear and tear will happen, causing pain, movement challenges, and a weak core. When people think of strengthening their core, they simply imagine doing more planks or crunches, but if their core is not functioning optimally, then all the planks in the world will do nothing for it and in fact will do more harm than good. Our increasingly sedentary lifestyle actually sets us up for a dysfunctional core, between all the sitting we do and all the high-intensity exercise we pursue (to make up for all the sitting we do). When you add pregnancy and birth onto those, the dysfunction is simply exaggerated.

Pregnancy and childbirth greatly affect your posture and alignment, and, therefore your breathing and core function, but by learning proper alignment and preventive exercise during pregnancy, you can help minimize the negative effects and keep your core strong and functional. The coolest thing is that many of the preventive Prepare To Push™ exercises you do during pregnancy are also the restorative exercises you will do postpartum, so you will already know what to do once your baby is born!

Let's look a bit more closely at the Core 4 so you gain a deeper understanding of how it works, how it supports you and your baby, and how you can best support it during pregnancy and as a new mom.

The Diaphragm

The diaphragm is a sheet of skeletal muscle that separates the heart, lungs, and ribs (the thoracic cavity) from the abdominal cavity. The diaphragm is convex in shape and is involved in breathing—it contracts and relaxes with each inhale and exhale. When you inhale, the diaphragm concentrically contracts as it lowers, pulling air in. Think of your abdominal cavity as a cylinder filling up with air and expanding as the air moves in. When you exhale, the fibres of the diaphragm eccentrically contract (lengthen) as it rises back to its resting state, emptying the air from the cylinder. In a well-functioning core, the pelvic floor (the diaphragm's BFF) will move along with the diaphragm during each inhalation and exhalation. As the diaphragm contracts, the pelvic floor expands and lengthens. As the diaphragm lengthens, the pelvic floor contracts and lifts.

The Transversus Abdominis

The deepest abdominal layer is the transversus abdominis (TVA), which runs around you like a corset and is a key muscle for pushing your baby out. It also plays an important role in stabilizing the lower back and pelvis before movement—yes, *before!* The TVA (and the entire core, for that matter) should anticipate and prepare you for movement without you even thinking about it. When the core is dysfunctional, it loses this ability to anticipate and can set you up for back or pelvic pain.

The movement of the TVA is inward, toward the spine, on the exhale and outward, away from the spine, on the inhale. A good point to remember is that in an ideally functioning core, the TVA co-contracts with the pelvic floor: on the exhale, the pelvic floor contracts and lifts while the belly moves inward, and on the inhale, the pelvic floor and belly expand. This is the foundation of the core breath, coming up in chapter 4. Your takeaway here is that the pelvic floor and the TVA co-contract and this synergy plays a key role preventing and healing mummy tummy!

The Pelvic Floor

Your pelvic floor is a group of muscles, in three layers, that run from the pubic bone (which is actually a joint called the pubic symphysis) to the tailbone, as well as the sitz bones (the ischial tuberosities). The pelvic floor is highly vascular (meaning it has a large blood supply), as well as highly innervated (it has a lot of nerves). The nerves, muscles, and connective tissue work to keep you continent, to provide support to your internal organs (the bladder, the uterus, and the rectum), to stabilize your spine and pelvis, and to contribute to your sexual satisfaction.

The pelvic floor also plays a major role in childbirth. But because it is not visible, the pelvic floor is rarely thought of until there's a problem, and then, because it plays such a central role in so much of what you do, it becomes the *only* thing you think about. Problems with the pelvic floor will often show up during pregnancy or after childbirth—problems such as incontinence, pelvic pain, organ prolapse, sexual challenges, back pain, and hip pain. These problems, collectively known as *pelvic floor dysfunction,* can develop from a variety of reasons, such as overuse (muscles that don't relax and that are tight and weak as a result), underuse (muscles that lack tone and are weak), injury (perineal or nerve injury from birth, sports, accidents, or surgeries), or poor posture and alignment. These problems are often preventable with the right information, alignment, and movement, but unfortunately, the pelvic floor is too often overlooked during a time when it is most at risk. The pelvic floor is the foundation of your core, and it deserves a lot more attention than it gets!

The Multifidus

The multifidus muscles are a group of short muscles located on both sides of your spine, running from your tailbone, or sacrum, all the way up to your neck. They function to support and protect your spine. Weakness in this muscle group contributes to chronic, dull low back pain. That pain, in turn, can inhibit these muscles from functioning, so they then become weak which creates a vicious pain–weakness cycle. The multifidus muscles are often overlooked in conditioning programs, which can result in these muscles needing to work extra hard to avoid back injury and compensate for weak abdominals.

The Core 4

Your core, when working optimally, is like a well-oiled machine: each part has its role and does its job. When the body is aligned, all of the parts of the core do their job naturally. The exercises in the Prepare to Push™ program start with alignment and incorporate breathing and movement. They require the Core 4 to work together as a team so that you can eliminate the aches and pains most women think are normal during pregnancy and as a new mom.

Now that you have a deeper understanding of what the true core really is, let's look at how pregnancy and birth can affect its function. This will allow you to take steps in your pregnancy and birth to avoid the common types of dysfunction that many people suffer with and think are normal.

CHAPTER TWO

How Pregnancy & Birth (& Life!) Can Affect Your Core

Pregnancy and birth are miraculous, and often our marvel at this miracle makes it easy to forget that it is a very physical event that can really take a toll on the body. As natural as it is, pregnancy and childbirth can leave the body in an injured state. But with the right information and preparation, injury can be minimized and recovery optimized.

Posture, hormones, number of babies, size of babies, number of pregnancies, vaginal birth, C-sections... these all affect your body, and can cause some things to not work as they used to. Many women wait until they are "done having kids" to "fix" their bodies and while it is never too late, waiting means you have a much bigger recovery hill to climb. **By being proactive, you will be able to prevent or minimize the issues that are commonly associated with pregnancy and birth and be in a better position to get back to the body you want.** Let's look at some of the more common aspects of pregnancy and birth that can contribute to core challenges.

Pregnancy

The abdominal wall, pelvic floor, and low back undergo increasing strain with the weight of the growing baby, the expanding uterus, and the additional fluids. Adding to this strain is the effect of the hormones on ligament laxity, making the joints less stable. These changes all contribute to alterations in your posture that can affect your alignment, and therefore the function of your core and surrounding muscles. The pelvis will often start to tip anteriorly, the shoulders round as the breasts grow, and the head juts forward. Actually this forward head, rounded shoulders posture is the one most people live in all day, every day, without even being pregnant! Truth be told, many women actually start their pregnancy with elements of core dysfunction. Huh— who knew?!

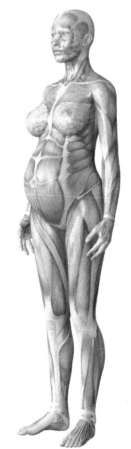

In pregnancy, the centre of gravity is shifting. Women try to counteract this forward shift in body weight by leaning back, pushing the hips forward, and clenching the butt muscles. The tailbone tucks and the hips thrust forward, and stability is then attempted by gripping in the butt, and the obliques. These are non-optimal strategies, and are the body's way of trying to stabilize itself when the muscles that should be supporting the core are not working properly because of poor posture and alignment. They are compensations, and they need to be prevented or changed. These poor core stability strategies alter the breathing and overuse the posterior pelvic floor and move the pelvic floor into a less supported position. They also inhibit and weaken the glutes and increase intra-abdominal pressure, which is not good news for the abdomen or the pelvic floor. Add to this the extra weight from the growing uterus, and you have a pelvic floor that is overworked *and* out of position! The good news is that even if you go into pregnancy with an element of core dysfunction, and even if you already have some aches and pains, you can take steps now to reverse them and prevent these things from becoming a bigger problem.

Fear

It may seem odd, but fear can affect your core and have a profound effect on your birth. One way it can affect your core is through a muscle called the psoas. The psoas runs from the spine through the pelvis to the upper leg and is the only muscle that joins the top and bottom parts of our bodies. This muscle (actually there are two psoas muscles—one on either side of the body) is typically tight because of the amount of sitting we do and the postures we live in. A tight psoas can pull on the spine, which changes our alignment. And because it runs through the pelvis, a tight psoas can also limit the amount of space in the pelvis for a baby to move into. This can lead to carrying the baby farther out front, which can cause more strain on the abdominal wall.

Fear can also cause this muscle to be tense. During labour, when you are trying to create the easiest transition for your baby with an "open door" to the world, you need the psoas muscles to be free of fear and tension so that your baby can navigate into and out of the pelvis.

The second way fear can impact your core is through your pelvic floor. Fear can cause you to hold on to tension in your pelvic floor, which can result in chronically contracted muscles, a tucked-under tailbone, and pelvic pain. Just as you need the psoas to relax, you also need your pelvic floor to be able to relax and let go of tension. By holding tension in the muscles of the pelvic floor, you can reduce the space for your baby and "close the door." leading to a more difficult time during labour.

This may all seem like a lot of doom and gloom, but it is meant to move you to action—action you will take in order to prepare and prevent! Going through pregnancy and birth armed with this knowledge puts you in a position of power. You can make informed decisions during your pregnancy, your birth, *and* your postpartum recovery, decisions that put you in the driver's seat rather than leave you just hoping for the best.

Now that we have looked at how pregnancy, birth, and life can affect your core, let's delve deeper into the two main aspects of the core that are left out of many prenatal education classes: the abdomen and the pelvic floor.

Childbirth

Childbirth, whether vaginal or surgical, can greatly affect the core. Vaginal birth causes extensive strain on the pelvic floor muscles, connective tissue, and nerves. This alters the pelvic landscape which can affect the overall feel and function of the pelvic floor. Even in the absence of tearing or an episiotomy, dysfunction can occur due to the excessive pressure, stretch, and compression that take place during the first and second stages of labour. Many women also face other interventions that increase the potential of tearing and episiotomy—interventions such as forceps, vacuum extraction, and prolonged pushing in the second stage of labour. The act of pushing can also stress the abdominal wall and if diastasis recti has not already occurred in pregnancy, it may occur during the pushing phase of labour. By following the guidelines in Prepare to Push™, you will go into birth knowing how to push and how to optimize your labour so that you will be less likely to face a prolonged second stage of labour, a "stalled" labour, or interventions.

A surgical birth, or cesarean section, involves incisions into the abdominal wall and the uterus which alters everything—the ligaments, the organs, the muscles, the tissues. A cesarean birth, while it may offer a small protective affect with regards to pelvic organ prolapse (more on that later) changes the body and leaves

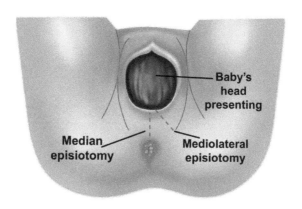

Median
episiotomy

Baby's
head
presenting

Mediolateral
episiotomy

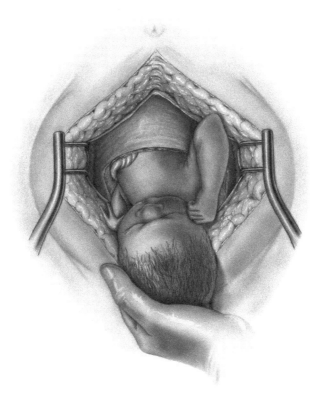

behind multiple layers of adhesions that can become the cause of pain and dysfunction. And keep in mind, a cesarean birth or C-section, does not make you immune to core dysfunction—in fact, in many cases it can leave you even more compromised. You have faced the same hormonal and postural changes in pregnancy, along with the weight of the baby on the pelvic floor throughout the pregnancy, and many women who have C-sections have gone into labour and pushed before ending up with a surgical birth! Learning proper healing techniques for both vaginal and Caesarean births can help prevent or minimize the likelihood of long-term challenges.

Breastfeeding

Who knew that breastfeeding could have an impact on core function? During pregnancy, breasts become enlarged, which can contribute to alterations in posture and alignment. Even without pregnancy and birth, slouching has become a typical posture for us in our computer-driven world, and once breastfeeding starts, you will live in that posture even more. Paying extra attention to posture and alignment during pregnancy and then as you start breastfeeding is key! This program will help you identify how to stand, sit, and move with your core well aligned.

Diastasis Recti

During pregnancy, the outermost abdominal muscles (the rectus abdominis) become stretched and weak and will start to move away from the midline—the linea alba—which also thins and stretches. This means less support for the spine and pelvis under the increasing load of pregnancy. This stretching of the muscles and connective tissue is a normal part of pregnancy (to an extent): it is how your body adjusts to accommodate the growing uterus and baby. But it can be made much worse by poor alignment, posture and exercise and it can certainly wreak havoc on the function of the core. When the muscles are stretched beyond their

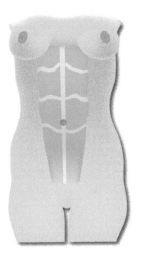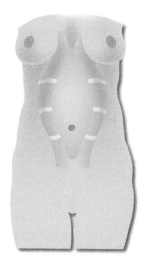

optimal length, which they clearly are in pregnancy, it means they don't work as they should. This in turn means back pain, pelvic pain, and ineffective pushing when it comes time to birth your baby. The good news is that with the right posture and alignment, and by choosing the right preventive exercise, this havoc can be minimized. More on this in the next chapter.

Postpartum Return to Exercise

Many women want nothing more than to get back into their regular clothes and resume or start a fitness program as soon as possible after delivery, so they can lose the baby weight and feel like themselves again. But desperately needed core restoration is unfortunately not even a consideration for most, and a premature return to high-impact exercise such as running, intense workouts, and the endless of crunches in the neighbourhood mommy boot camp do far more harm than good. The first eight weeks postpartum are critical to healing. Knowing what to do and what to avoid during this time will ensure that you can get back to the activities you want with a body you are confident in. Your doctor or midwife will see you for a six-week postpartum checkup to ensure that your uterus has returned to its non-pregnant state. This is typically when he/she gives you the green light to get back to your regular activities. In my opinion, this is irresponsible. While the uterus may have shrunk back to its original size, the pelvis and abdomen are nowhere near ready for a return to regular activities. Consider the six-week checkup as your green light to go see your pelvic floor physiotherapist for a thorough assessment of your core and pelvic floor function, and please refrain from registering for the mom-and-baby classes until your core is restored (which can take 4–6 months or more). My slogan is "*Mommy* and *boot camp* do not belong in the same sentence."

Previous Injuries

Old injuries, surgeries, strains, and sprains from life as an adventurous child, or involvement in sports, or car accidents— can all cause compensations and leave your core more vulnerable to new strains, such as those from pregnancy and birth. When you start with non-optimal strategies that have developed from previous injuries and then add the stress and strain from pregnancy and birth, you can end up in an even more disadvantaged position. The preventive exercises in this book, combined with visits to a pelvic floor physiotherapist during your pregnancy, will help you feel better and stronger before your baby is born and may even help get rid of the nagging issues you thought you had to live with!

CHAPTER THREE

Mummy Tummy (Diastasis Recti) & Pelvic Floor Dysfunction

The Two Most Common Types of Core Dysfunction That No One Tells You About!

Let's be honest: most women are concerned about how big their belly will get and if it will ever be the same once the baby is born. Most are proud to show off their belly once they start to show, but as their belly gets bigger and bigger, thoughts turn to stretch marks and to wondering if it will ever look the same again.

For such an obvious change to the body, it is amazing that more attention has not been paid to what is actually happening to the muscles and connective tissue in the abdomen and what the impact of these changes actually means. Women deserve to know more, and *should* know more, so they can take steps to minimize the impact of pregnancy and birth on their bodies.

Diastasis Recti, a.k.a. Mummy Tummy—a Deeper Look

One of the most common complaints of women after they have had a baby is their tummy. "How do I get my tummy back to the way it used to be?" "I just want this pooch to go away." "I look six months' pregnant all the time!"

As mentioned earlier, diastasis recti, or mummy tummy, as it is often referred to, occurs when the connective tissue that holds in place the two rectus muscles (the six-pack muscles) thins and weakens, which results in the muscles moving away from the midline, their optimal alignment. This separation can happen from your sternum all the way down to your pubic joint, which is a pretty big distance! Generally, it's worst at the belly button. Some women may have it *only* at their belly button, while others can have it along the entire length of the abdomen. When the muscles aren't in the proper alignment, they aren't able to work as well as they should. This is one way that compensations and non-optimal strategies for movement and stability start to develop. When one part of the core is compromised so that it can't do its job, something else has to step in and pick up the slack.

Everyone focuses on the separation, or the distance between the two rectus muscles, which is fair given that the term *diastasis recti* means "separation" of the "rectus muscles," but it is not the separation that is actually the main problem (other than aesthetics)—rather, it's the loss of integrity in the connective tissue. This point is overlooked in most diastasis assessments and recovery programs. Most programs focus on closing the separation and don't pay any attention to the connective tissue underneath. The truth is, many times the muscles themselves actually do not realign completely, if at all, yet if the linea alba is able to generate tension, then the core can be supported and considered "functional." While closing the gap may be considered ideal, we need to pay more attention to the connective tissue—the linea alba. In order for the linea alba to heal, the core needs to be in optimal alignment, and the Core 4 needs to be working together, at rest and when moving. By using the exercises in this book to prepare, and then again to restore postpartum, you will minimize the diastasis and you will also harness the most optimal healing time (the first eight weeks postpartum) and so will be more likely to see your muscles realign *and* the connective tissue recover and be able to generate the tension required for core stability.

If you've already had a pregnancy in which you had a diastasis and it never healed properly, when you get pregnant again, the already stretched and weak muscles are now under more strain and you are likely to show sooner. Women can show as early as twelve or thirteen weeks in subsequent pregnancies when perhaps it was closer to four or five months previously. Having an existing diastasis can also contribute to back pain and as mentioned earlier, can influence your ability to push successfully during labour, so it is important to take steps to prevent it as well as heal it in between pregnancies.

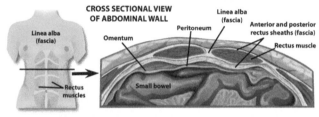

NORMAL ABDOMINAL WALL ANATOMY

CROSS SECTIONAL VIEW OF ABDOMINAL WALL

Linea alba (fascia)

Peritoneum

Anterior and posterior rectus sheaths (fascia)

Linea alba (fascia)

Omentum

Rectus muscle

Rectus muscles

Small bowel

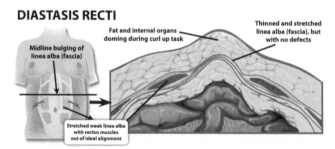

DIASTASIS RECTI

Fat and internal organs doming during curl up task

Thinned and stretched linea alba (fascia), but with no defects

Midline bulging of linea alba (fascia)

Stretched weak linea alba with rectus muscles out of ideal alignment

Healing a Diastasis

The first eight weeks postpartum are the most critical in terms of healing the connective tissue and encouraging the rectus muscles to realign. If you can harness those first eight weeks by supporting the tissues with a belly wrap and restoring the core from the inside out with appropriate exercise, you will be less likely to suffer from the most common types of core dysfunction. By preparing to push, you will maintain a stronger core in pregnancy, which will help you avoid or minimize diastasis; you will be more effective at pushing; and you will regain your form and function much more quickly and easily after your baby is born.

A product I recommend for helping heal diastasis recti is the AB Tank by Bellies Inc. (Full disclosure: I am a partner in the business and helped design and develop the product.) It is designed to provide light compressive support to the healing tissues while also encouraging the displaced abdominal muscles to realign. It is meant to be put on immediately after giving birth (so you want to purchase it while you are still pregnant!) and is meant to be used in conjunction with restorative exercise.

Ultimately, it is easier to prepare and prevent than it is to try to fix things once they have happened. Often, health care professionals will say, "We'll fix it once you're done having children." But waiting means the hill is much bigger to climb. By addressing the issue preventatively during your pregnancy and then taking steps to restore form and function in the early weeks postpartum, you will be less likely to suffer from mummy tummy or pelvic floor dysfunction.

Pelvic Floor Dysfunction

When functioning optimally, the pelvic floor helps support your spine and pelvis, it holds your internal organs in place, it helps keep you continent, and it contributes to sexual satisfaction. Unfortunately, as we have discussed, pregnancy and birth can negatively affect the ideal function of the pelvic floor and can contribute to some common types of pelvic floor dysfunction. Notice I said "common," not "normal." Back pain, pelvic pain, tearing, incontinence, diastasis recti, organ prolapse, and unsatisfying sex—these things are often thought of as normal once you become pregnant or after you have a baby. The truth is, while they are common, they are not normal, and they don't have to be a part of your pregnancy or postpartum experience. Health care professionals might say, "These are just part of being pregnant," but that's not true. You have the power to do things differently and to prepare your body for birth and recovery. The Prepare to Push™ program trains your muscles specifically for pregnancy and birth to keep them functioning optimally.

The pelvic floor is often not really thought about until a woman becomes pregnant, and even then not so much. After the baby is born, when things don't feel right, it is the *only* thing a woman can think about, but because it is embarrassing or she thinks this experience is normal, she suffers in silence.

Thoughts about the pelvic floor in pregnancy usually are along the lines of "How am I going to get this baby out, and will I still be able to hold a tampon in?" "Will I still enjoy sex? Will my partner still enjoy it?" "Will I pee my pants when I exercise?" These are all valid concerns, and by thinking about them during pregnancy, you are more likely to take steps to prevent and maintain your pelvic floor wellness. The good news is that the body is designed to give birth, and that with the information, awareness, and preparation you will gain from this book, you will support your body and set yourself up for a better birth and recovery that has you still enjoying sex, keeping a tampon in, and not leaking!

A deeper understanding of the pelvic floor and what it actually goes through in pregnancy and birth can help prepare you both mentally and physically for the big day. Seeing a pelvic floor physiotherapist during and after your pregnancy (and then once a year after that) is an ideal way to prevent and treat pelvic floor dysfunction.

Pelvic floor challenges can result from overuse or underuse of the muscles. Your muscles have been working hard through your pregnancy to try to maintain stability in your pelvis, maintain stability in your spine, keep your organs in place, and manage the ever-increasing load of the growing baby—all this while trying to maintain your continence and your sex life too! When muscles overwork, they can become weak, because they never get a break. The reason they become overused is that they are trying to pick up the slack from other muscles that are not able to do their job because of posture or alignment changes.

Here are some of the more common types of pelvic floor dysfunction and tips on how to prevent them or treat them.

Incontinence

One common side effect of pregnancy and delivery (notice again that I said "common" and not "normal") is incontinence—the involuntary loss of urine.

There are a few different types of incontinence. *Stress incontinence* occurs if you are exerting a force like running, laughing, coughing, sneezing, or jumping and urine leaks out a little bit at a time. *Urge incontinence* is when you feel like you have to go all the time, or like you can't hold it, and you can't make it to the bathroom in time. *Mixed incontinence* is a combination of stress and urge incontinence. Incontinence can occur as a result of nerve damage or scar tissue, from overused muscles, and from underused muscles, but the good news is that it can be prevented and treated with alignment, breath work and pelvic muscle exercise, ideally with a pelvic floor physiotherapist, before and after birth.

Pelvic Organ Prolapse

Pelvic organ prolapse is a challenge that is even less known and talked about than incontinence. Yet 50% of women who have had children will have some degree of prolapse, most unaware of it due to the few symptoms this condition has in the early stages. Also, 50% of women who have diastasis recti will have some element of pelvic floor dysfunction (mainly incontinence and prolapse). Of note here is that prolapse does not occur only in women who have had children. Pregnancy and birth increase the risk, but prolapse can happen in women who have never been pregnant or had children, pointing to other influences such as posture, lifestyle, age, and hormones.

As noted earlier, one of the functions of the pelvic floor is to help keep the pelvic organs in place. The positions of the bladder, the uterus, and the rectum are partially dependent on the strength and position of the pelvis and pelvic floor muscles. A weakened

Rectum

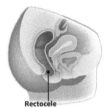

Rectocele

Normal
Female Pelvic Anatomy

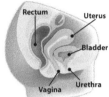

Rectum
Uterus
Bladder
Vagina
Urethra

Cystocele Prolapse

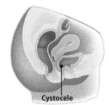

Cystocele

Normal
Female Pelvic Anatomy

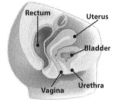

Rectum
Uterus
Bladder
Vagina
Urethra

Uterine Prolapse

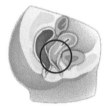

Normal
Female Pelvic Anatomy

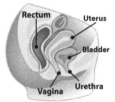

Rectum
Uterus
Bladder
Vagina
Urethra

Vaginal Vault Prolapse

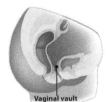

Vaginal vault

Normal
Female Pelvic Anatomy
(post-hysterectomy)

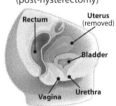

Rectum
Uterus
(removed)
Bladder
Vagina
Urethra

pelvic floor loses its ability to provide support, which can interfere with the ability to hold the organs in their anatomical positions. Unsupported organs will start to descend into and, in severe cases, out of the vagina, which is obviously something you want to avoid. There are four stages of prolapse: early stage prolapse, grades 1 and 2, is often asymptomatic, which is why your preventive pelvic floor physiotherapist visits are such a key part of your health care team. When caught at grade 1 or 2, prolapse can be well managed and may even be reversed. Grade 3 occurs when the organ is at the introitus (the entrance to the vagina), and grade 4 occurs when the organ is bulging out of the vagina. Once the organ, or organs—you can have more than one organ prolapsing—get down close to the opening of the vagina or out of the vagina, there is no reversing that: it typically calls for surgery. Prolapse is not life-threatening, but it is *very* life-altering. Many young women living with prolapse will say, "My body is broken" and "Why didn't anyone tell me this could happen?" With the right information and preparation, prolapse does not have to be part of your postpartum body.

Pelvic Girdle Pain
Symphysis Pubis Dysfunction

One common challenge that can present in pregnancy is pain in the pubic joint. A lot of women report feeling as though they have been kicked in the crotch. They might find it hard to stand on one leg to put pants on, and it might be challenging to roll over in bed or to get in and out of a car. Pain in the pubic joint is called *symphysis pubis dysfunction*. In pregnancy, the pubic joint starts to widen, loosen, and become more lax in preparation for baby. As a result, the pelvis can become less stable and can cause pain at that joint.

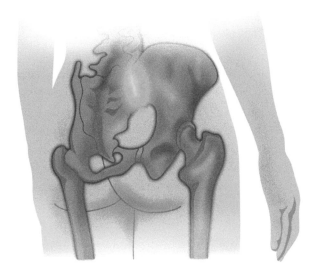

A very common location of pain in pregnancy is the sacroiliac, or SI, joint, where the sacrum meets the iliac bones. Note, there are two joints—one on either side—and the pain can be in one or both sides... and can be very debilitating. The postural changes in pregnancy can affect this joint, the hormones making the pelvis more "open" can affect this joint, the added weight on the pelvis can affect this joint, and weak or compromised pelvic floor muscles can affect this joint.

During pregnancy, as many as 42% of women will have some form of pelvic pain, with sacroiliac (SI joint) and symphysis pubis pain being the most common. Wearing a support belt like the BabyBellyBand or the Baby Belly Belt during and after pregnancy can provide relief and help stabilize the pelvis while function is restored through alignment and exercise. Pelvic floor exercise is critical as it will help strengthen the muscles that support the pelvis and help release the muscles that may be overworking or compensating for weakness elsewhere.

Scar Tissue

Another pelvic floor challenge that can occur as a result of labour and delivery results from scar tissue. You can end up with scar tissue on the labia and perineum from tearing or if you have an episiotomy and if you have a surgical birth, you would have abdominal scar tissue. Scar tissue creates adhesions as the tissue heals, which is natural and needed, but you want to keep the adhesions as mobile as possible so that they don't stick to places you don't want and start to cause movement restrictions.

Fascia is thin, white connective tissue that we all have in our body. It is a system that envelops muscle but it also interconnects between the muscles. When you have an incision or injury, the connective tissue starts to create adhesions. A restriction (from adhesions) in the connective tissue can actually create pain in another part of the body as it pulls muscles or organs out of their optimal positions. Avoiding perineal tearing or episiotomy is obviously ideal, but working postpartum with a pelvic floor physiotherapist who can mobilize the scar tissue once it has occurred is a must!

***

Okay—enough of the heavy stuff. Let's look at how you can prevent and prepare so you can avoid all of this trouble!

CHAPTER FOUR

Prevent Dysfunction & Restore Function with the Core Breath

Okay, so that last chapter was a bit heavy. However, it is important to know these things ahead of time so you can be proactive, take steps to prevent and also know who to see and how to best recover once your baby is born. By preparing to push you are taking control, and putting yourself in a position of power, armed with information!

The Core Breath

Mummy tummy and pelvic floor dysfunction, along with back pain and unsatisfying sex, seem to be considered normal after having children, leading most women to think they need to learn to live with it while suffering in silence. These conditions are common but not normal, and with the right information and training, these aspects of core dysfunction can be prevented or minimized so that you can get through birth in one piece and enjoy motherhood. By connecting with your core during pregnancy, you can better support your body through the inevitable changes, perform better during labour, and optimize your postpartum recovery. To help you connect with your core, I will teach you what I call the *core breath*.

You are probably asking yourself why you need to be taught how to breathe—you've been doing it since you were born, right? Well, we all have, but life can cause our breathing patterns to change. How we sit, how we stand, how we move and how often we move, the activities we pursue, injuries, surgeries—these and more can all affect how we breathe. And if our breathing is not as it should be, then neither is our core. Yes, your breath affects your core! The cool part about the core breath is that it is both preventive (you will use it throughout you pregnancy to help maintain your core function) and restorative (it is the first exercise you will do to help restore form and function after your baby is born). This functional breath encourages better alignment and posture and allows you to connect with your core during pregnancy, during birth, and as a new mom. Talk about mind/body birth prep!

Connecting with your core all starts with the breath. Actually, it all starts with alignment and *then* the breath, because if you aren't in optimal alignment, you can't breathe properly, and then the core is not set up for ideal function. So let's talk about alignment. Whether you are standing or sitting, your pelvis should live underneath the ribs, your tailbone should be untucked, and there should be a gentle curve in your low back. Here is a great example of poor vs. great alignment in pregnancy, courtesy of Susanne Reinhold of Kangaroo Fitness in Ottawa, Ontario.

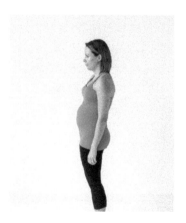 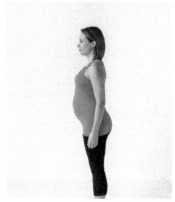

In the first image here, you can see how the woman's hips are pressed forward and her upper back is behind her pelvis. Nothing is lined up, meaning her core is not in the optimal position. In the second photo, everything lines up as it should, meaning her core is able to work. Whether standing or sitting, your core needs to be lined up in order to function as it should.

So the first step in learning the core breath is to make sure your core is lined up. Use a mirror and practise standing and sitting in alignment. I suggest starting seated on a stability ball or birth ball because the roundness of the ball provides great feedback on the perineum regarding what is happening in the pelvic floor. Here are step-by-step instructions:

- Sit on your ball and pull your bum flesh out from under you so that you can really feel your perineum on the ball and are aware of your sitz bones.

- Look in the mirror beside you so that you can see yourself. Find the gentle curve in the low back and the position of the pelvis in relation to the rib cage. Your feet will be flat on the floor and slightly wider than pelvis-width apart.

- Now put one hand on your belly and one hand on your ribs. Breathe into your hands... Inhale to expand.

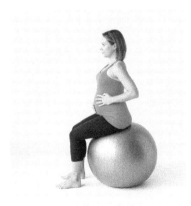

Inhale to Expand

You should feel your ribs expand and your belly expand as the air draws in and fills you up. The goal is to get the breath into the ribs and into the belly. For some people, it helps to think about breathing sideways, to bring the air to your ribs. For others it helps to visualize inflating a balloon inside you. Watch yourself in the mirror and see where your breath goes: Do your shoulders lift? Does your stomach move inward as you inhale? These are signs of reverse breathing. It may take some practice to get it right, but keep at it! Once you have it, just focus on the inhale for a while—inhale to expand feel your ribs inflate and your belly expand, and bring your awareness to your pelvic floor. Feel space between your sitz bones and a sense of fullness in your perineum. You can visit pelviennewellness.com and find a full video on the core breath.

Focus just on the in-breath for a while, and really connect with the feeling of expansion that each inhale brings to your ribs, your belly, and your pelvic floor.

The diaphragm moves down as you breathe in and up as you breathe out. The pelvic floor works in synergy with the diaphragm, so it also descends (expands) as you breathe in and lifts (contracts) as you breathe out.

You've connected with the inhale; now bring your awareness to your exhale. As your breathe out, feel the ribs soften, the belly move inward, and the pelvic floor lift. You may feel less fullness in your perineum and less space between the sitz bones, and have less awareness of the surface of the ball. (The roundness of the ball can help with the changing sensations in the pelvic floor, but if you feel like you aren't quite getting it, try moving into a wide-leg child's pose. (See the image on page 74. For some, this pose works really well for truly "feeling" the breath and where it goes.) Once you've connected with the out-breath, I want you to purse your lips and blow, as if you are blowing out birthday candles—a slow, audible exhale through pursed lips. How did that change the sensations? Were you more aware of the movement in your pelvic floor? By pursing your lips, you change the sensations of pressure and heighten the sensation of lift and inward movement of the pelvic floor and belly. Notice in the photo below, the position of the belly in relation to the hand. The lips are pursed and the pelvic floor engaging, which is causing a co-contraction of the deep abdominals, which then move inward toward the spine. Think of it as a gentle lift (from the pelvic floor) and hug (from the transversus abdominis) for your baby.

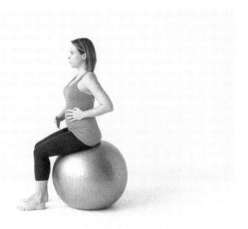

This is the core breath: Inhale to Expand, Exhale to Engage. Always exhale through pursed lips and add in your voluntary pelvic floor contraction. Now for the fun part— you can add in some visualizations to really connect with the lifting movement of the pelvic floor.

One of my favourite visualizations is to imagine a jellyfish swimming to the surface of the ocean. As you breathe in, visualize the jellyfish floating softly and freely in the water. As you purse

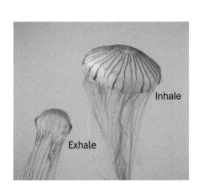

your lips and exhale, visualize the edges of the jellyfish coming together and the jellyfish propelling itself to the surface. In this case, your perineum is the jellyfish— open, soft and free on the inhale, closed and propelling up toward the crown of the head on the exhale.

Here are some other visualizations to try... Imagine, as you exhale, that you

- are preventing a tampon from slipping out
- are sipping a milkshake through a straw with your vagina
- are picking up a blueberry with your vagina and anus
- are pulling your partner's finger or penis deeper into you
- are lifting your perineum up toward the crown of your head
- have a drawstring attached to your sitz bones, your tailbone, and your pubic bone, and are cinching the drawstring and lifting it up toward the crown of your head

Try them all and see which one resonates most with you, then stick with that one each time your practice your core breath and anytime someone asks you to engage your core. If jellyfish *is* your best cue, then your core breath would be this:

Inhale to expand, feeling space and softness in your perineum as the jellyfish floats softly. Purse your lips and blow as you exhale to engage and propel the jellyfish upward to the surface of the ocean.

Each time you inhale, you are relaxing and softening the pelvic floor as it expands. Each time you exhale, you are voluntarily lifting and engaging your pelvic floor as it contracts.

Core breathing supports the optimal function of your core and naturally strengthens the pelvic floor, the multifidus and the deep abdominals. By practising daily throughout your pregnancy, you will maintain a fit and healthy core while preventing or minimizing diastasis recti and pelvic floor challenges.

The core breath will also come into play in labour and birth (with a slight modification I will teach you later). Core breathing is also the very first restorative exercise you will do postpartum and should be started as soon as possible after birth (I don't mean minutes after, but within a day or two is ideal). Using the core breath restoratively helps the mind/body connection, helps restore tone and function to the pelvic floor and deep abdominals, encourages blood flow to the healing tissues, and, by gently working the pelvic floor muscles, also promotes healing of any nerve damage that may have taken place.

What about Kegels?

Kegel exercises are very well intended, but they are a static exercise that is trying to isolate one muscle, plus most people focus only on the contraction and not on the relaxation. Core breathing is a functional, dynamic exercise that uses voluntary contractions and releases of the pelvic floor—much more effective than doing kegels at every red light! (Truth be told, Kegels are actually less effective if you do them seated in the car given the poor pelvic alignment that car seats put you in.)

If you are unable to feel yourself contracting and releasing your pelvic floor, then it is best to seek the help of your pelvic floor physiotherapist, who will teach you to actively contract and relax your pelvic floor and will determine what may be interfering with your ability to sense the movement in the muscles.

Here are a few more tips. Try thinking about lifting your vagina into your abdomen (you can also use your own fingers to help feel this). If you have an EPI-NO (see chapter 6), it is a great tool to help you connect with your pelvic floor contractions and, more importantly, your ability to let go of those contractions! What you're trying to feel for when you contract is a sense of closure of the openings (the vagina, rectum and urethra), and a lift. It's not just about squeezing as hard as you can, but rather about a gentle inward and upward lift. When you are letting go, you want to feel a sense of release and softening—a sense of space and openness.

During pregnancy, you can practise your core breath on the stability ball, but in the early weeks postpartum, even if there was no tearing, the pressure of the ball will be uncomfortable on the perineum, so choose a crook-lying or side-lying position or a supported wide-leg child's pose to practise. Keep in mind, side-lying is a great position for breastfeeding, so you can core breathe while nourishing your new babe.

The core breath keeps your core functioning optimally throughout your pregnancy, and it helps you return to optimal function postpartum. The best part about learning this during your pregnancy is that you won't have to learn something new in the postpartum period when you are working on lack of sleep, learning to breastfeed, and feeling overwhelmed by all of the other new things!

We've looked at how alignment and the core breath can help prevent some of the more common postpartum complaints. Now let's look at how you can optimize your birth by choosing birth positions that will facilitate your baby's arrival.

CHAPTER FIVE

Optimal Labour &
Birth Positions

When it comes to birth, the image most people have is of the woman lying on her back with her feet in stirrups and legs spread apart, the doctor at the vulva and a nurse at her head telling her when to push and then counting to 10 as the woman holds her breath and clenches her jaw while bearing down. This is the image you see on TV and in the movies, and is the experience your mother most likely had and that even some of your friends have had. Here's a little secret... This is the worst position to birth in! This position limits the space in your pelvis by restricting the movement of the sacrum, and it takes out the influence of gravity, so it is almost like you are pushing your baby up a hill through a tunnel! You have to push longer and harder, and there is more opportunity for damage to the tissues and for interventions.

Birth position can play a huge role in your birth outcome and in the length of time that you spend pushing. You want to keep the pushing phase under two hours—in fact, under an hour is even better! The longer the pushing time, the higher the likelihood of nerve damage due to the stretch, compression, and pressure and the more likely you will end up with interventions or even a C-section.

Sometimes women think that if they have a C-section, they avoid the negative consequences of vaginal birth and are therefore immune to pelvic floor problems. They fail to consider that they have had the same posture changes, hormonal influences, and weight of the baby on the pelvic floor during pregnancy. Many women go into labour then push for 2 hours, have interventions and *then* end up having a C-section. Even if a C-section is planned, there are multiple layers of adhesions through the abdomen, and this can sometimes compromise the core even more.

You want to limit the opportunities for intervention by changing birth positions as needed, by staying active and move in your labour, and by building a strong birth team—doula, midwife, pelvic floor physiotherapist, and prenatal/postpartum fitness professional.

There are many labour and birth positions that you can use. In early labour, it is important to try and stay upright and move around while keeping your pelvis free and mobile. Walk, sway, even dance! You will have gravity working for you, and moving your pelvis is important.

Here are some positions to try in early labour.

One Leg Standing

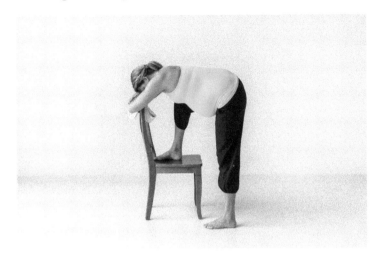

Standing is great for labour and birth as it uses gravity and keeps the pelvic outlet open and the sacrum free. By using a chair, a footstool, or a bench, you can raise one leg to alter the position of the pelvis as needed or as your comfort dictates to help your baby move down and out.

Bent-Over Supported

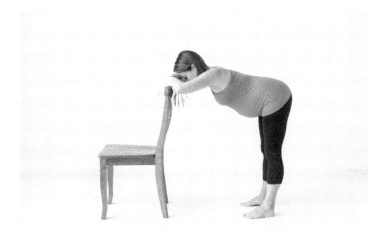

Standing and leaning forward can be very comforting during a contraction. This position is a great use of gravity while keeping the pelvis open and the sacrum free. It also allows for freedom of movement in the pelvis and allows you to sway and circle your pelvis, which can help you manage pain and help create space for the baby. Having a doula or partner behind you who can squeeze the pelvis (called the Hip Squeeze) can help relieve pain as well. You can also do this leaning over a couch or the hospital bed or even the kitchen counter.

Supported Seated

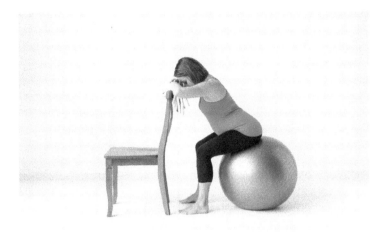

Sitting on the ball allows you to circle and rock your pelvis, which can help facilitate the movement of your baby into the pelvic outlet. Having a chair to lean forward on is very comforting and also allows for a doula or your partner to be behind you to place warm cloths on your neck, perform massage or acupressure or compress your pelvis (hips), which can feel fantastic during a contraction. You could also place the ball beside a couch, bed, or hospital bed so you have something to lean on. Your partner or birth professional can be someone to lean on as well.

Supported Squatting

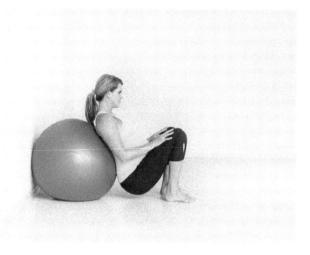

Squatting is great for labour. It keeps the body upright to harness the effects of gravity, and it keeps the pelvic outlet open to create space for your baby. For birth I prefer the supported squat as it reduces the stretch and strain on the perineum compared to the regular squat and also takes some of the load off the legs, which will be challenged! Supported squatting uses gravity, it keeps a nice open pelvis, and the sacrum is free. You can lean against a ball as pictured above, or back into the arms of your partner, or you can raise the back of your hospital bed and lean back. If you are at home, it could be the couch or a stack of pillows on your bed that you lean back onto. If you are in a birthing pool, place a chair near the outside edge and have your partner or doula sit on the chair with their feet in the water. You will squat in between their legs and drape your arms over their legs, or they can hold you under your arms.

Side-Lying

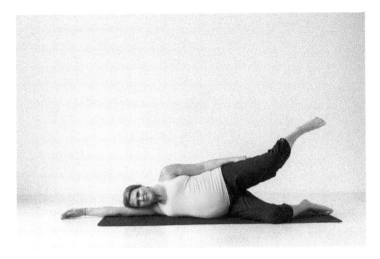

This is a great position to use if labour is progressing very rapidly. Taking out the effects of gravity can help slow things down while keeping the pelvic outlet open and the sacrum free. By turning the top knee slightly inward, you will open up the space between the sitz bones even more to create more space for your baby. Have your partner or doula hold your top leg for you. If you want to keep a bit of the influence of gravity, simply raise the top of the hospital bed slightly or use pillows, bolsters, or both to help elevate your upper body. This is also one of the positions that has been shown to be most likely to preserve the perineum.

All Fours

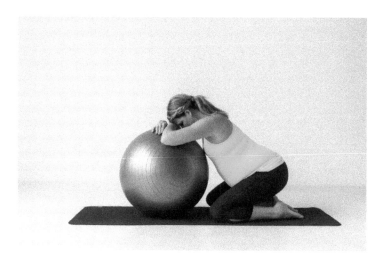

There are a lot of ways to be on all fours, and this is one of my favourites. You can do this as shown or you can modify it by taking the ball away and leaning forward into the thighs of your partner or birth professional. You can also do this in the birth pool, leaning over the edge with the chair or ball at the side of the pool. If you are at the hospital, raise the top of the hospital bed up and then turn and face it so you can drape your hands over the top and rest your head into the mattress.

***

By practising these birth positions ahead of time, you will build strength and endurance for the big day! You will also be familiar with what is comfortable for you and what modifications you would need according to where you are giving birth.

A great way to prepare your body for birth is to practise these positions during pregnancy and also choose exercises that mimic these birth positions. Check them out in the next chapter!

CHAPTER SIX

Prepare to Push™

Exercise for Birth

Now that we've looked at what birth positions are most favourable, we are going to look at what exercises you can do to prepare the muscles you will use in those birth positions. We will consider strength, endurance, and flexibility, as it is important to be strong, to have the endurance to manage labour and birth, and also to have muscles that can yield and release tension. The goals of the Prepare to Push™ program are to strengthen your core, increase space in the pelvis, strengthen the muscles of the hips, lengthen the calves, hamstrings and inner thighs, and prepare the pelvic floor.

Pelvic Rocking

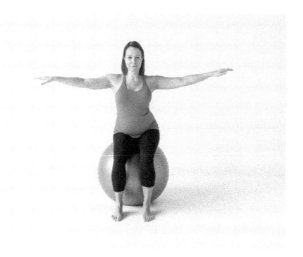

In the last chapter, I spoke a lot about rocking or circling the pelvis during labour to help facilitate the movement of your babe into the pelvis. By practising pelvic rocking during your pregnancy, you are building core strength, maintaining good mobility in your pelvis, and preparing your body for labour.

Sit on an exercise ball (though you can do this standing up if you don't have a ball, or if you prefer, you can belly dance!) with your arms out to the side for balance. This exercise is all about keeping mobility in your pelvis and giving your core a great workout. Try to keep your upper body fairly still and quiet while you dance your pelvis around on the ball: shift side to side, tuck under and release back, circle your pelvis one way and then the other, and then try figure 8s. The movement should be coming from your pelvis rather than your legs and upper body. Think hula hooper or belly dancer.

Once your baby is born, this exercise can be done around six to eight weeks postpartum after your perineum has healed. You will also find that your baby loves to be gently lulled to sleep while you circle and bounce on the ball.

The Bridge

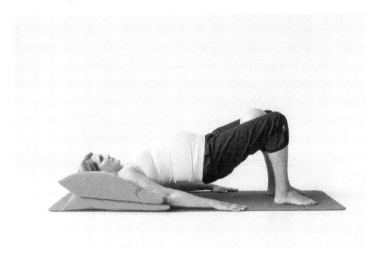

This is one of my favourite exercises of all time—such a great core exercise, and also one of the best glute builders around! During pregnancy, you can use a wedge or a stack of pillows under your head and shoulders to keep the heart above the pelvis, but if you feel okay on your back for 20–30 seconds, then you can do this without a wedge or pillows. Using a ball, a small pillow, or a yoga block between the thighs will help engage the inner thighs as well.

Now let's apply the core breath. Inhale to expand, then exhale to engage and press the hips up toward the ceiling. Inhale as you lower back down. Aim for 10–12 reps, 1–2 sets per day. **Note: If you have symphysis pubis dysfunction (SPD), perform the exercise without a ball or block between your legs.**

Postpartum, this will be one of the first exercises you do— usually around week 2. It is a great way to promote circulation in the healing core, it provides a gentle inversion to help the organs resume their optimal positions, and it helps restore pelvic stability.

The Clam

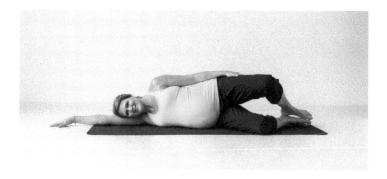

The clam is one of the classic core and pelvic floor exercises. Use it during pregnancy and in the early weeks postpartum. Remember the side-lying birth position? Well, the clam is an excellent exercise to practise for that position. This exercise helps strengthen the glutes, which are great pelvic floor supporters, and it will also help you hold your leg up.

Lie down on your side on a soft surface. Find your neutral pelvis, making sure there is a gentle curve in your low back, with your tailbone out from underneath you. Now add in your core breath: inhale to expand, and then exhale through pursed lips and engage the pelvic floor as you press your feet together and lift your top knee away from the bottom knee. Keep your feet pressed together the entire time and lift only as high as you can without your body starting to roll backward.

By adding the core breath to movement, you are building core strength and coordination and improving your overall core function. We are dynamic beings, so training our core through breath and movement mimics what we want and need our core to do in daily life. When you first start doing these exercises, you may feel a bit jerky, or maybe you won't feel like you can hold your pelvic floor contraction for very long, or maybe you will feel like you can't let go of the contraction. Don't worry—the more you do it, the smoother it will feel, and your endurance will build as well.

Postpartum, you will do the clam around week 3.

Broken Clam

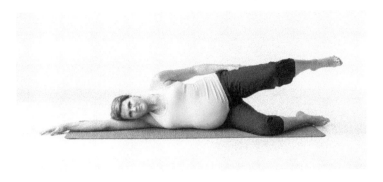

In the broken clam, the ankles are not pressed together but rather lift away from the bottom leg along with the knee. Your breath, however, stays the same. Inhale to expand, exhale to engage, then lift the top leg. Inhale as you lower the leg back down.

This exercise mimics the side-lying birth position even more closely than the regular clam, and you can play around with rotating your knee inward as you lift as well.

To get you even more in touch with your pelvis, try this: Start by lying on your left side and use your right hand to find your right sitz bone (the prominent bone that you feel deep in your butt cheek). Keep your fingers pressing on your right sitz bone. Now feel what happens when you rotate your knee. Bring your knee to point down toward the floor and then open it up to point up toward the ceiling. Can you feel how the space between your sitz bones closes and opens? Can you feel that with your knee pointing more upward, one sitz bone is closer to the other sitz bone? Can you feel that when you rotate your knee down toward the floor, it moves that sitz bone out of the way a little so they are farther apart? In the side-lying position, having your knee pointing down slightly actually creates more space in the pelvis for your baby during birth.

Feel around your pelvis with your hand. Can you find your pubic bone? Your tailbone? Put your hand on your low back and find your sacrum. Walk your fingertips down in between your bum cheeks and find your coccyx (tailbone). This bone is shaped like a triangle and needs to be able to move in labour. The tailbone naturally tucks and untucks as the baby moves down and out, so keeping the sacrum free during labour and birth is key. Now I want you to flip over onto your back. Can you see how giving birth in this position would restrict the movement of your sacrum and would keep your tailbone tucked the entire time? Not ideal for creating space for your baby! Lying on your back decreases the space in the pelvis, making it harder for the baby to move into it and out of it. Think about this for a second… When you need to go poo, do you go to the bathroom, lie down on the floor, and put your feet up? So why does it make sense to birth that way? Birth is an elimination, and being upright with an open pelvis helps elimination happen more freely.

The Wide Kneel

The wide kneel is preparing you for the kneeling and all fours birth positions. Take your knees about hip-width apart, or a little wider. (You may want to put some extra padding underneath your knees.) Your feet will be touching the ground behind you and your bum will be resting on your heels. Place your hands on your hips and inhale to expand. Now exhale to engage and then lift your bum away from your heels so you up come to a high kneel. Inhale as you lower back down to your heels.

During your pregnancy, you can place a stability ball or an ottoman in front of you to practise this with support.

Note: If you have symphysis pubis dysfunction (SPD), please avoid this exercise.

In the early weeks postpartum, being in a wide leg position can leave your pelvic floor feeling vulnerable, so you will add this in between six and eight weeks (if you feel okay with it), and you will start with a narrower stance and gradually progress to having the hips wider than the pelvis. If you feel any heaviness in your pelvis, pain in the pubic joint, or other discomfort, you can hold off on this exercise until you feel ready.

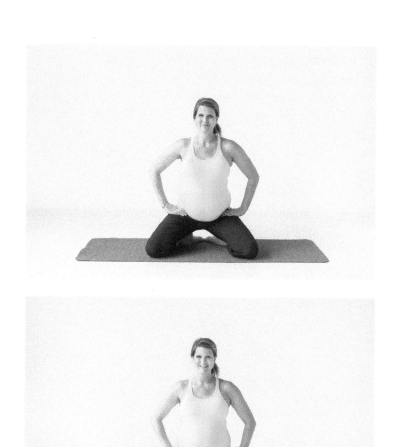

Squatting

This is a great exercise during your pregnancy, and it prepares you for squatting during labour. What it also does is prepare you for motherhood—you will be picking up your baby and putting your baby back down again several times a day, and squatting is the right way to do it. Once your children are bigger, you will be picking up and putting down an even heavier load. By building up strength and endurance in your pregnancy, you will have an easier time in birth *and* be set up for success in motherhood!

I like starting people, especially during pregnancy, with the ball between the back and the wall. Stand with your feet pelvis-width apart and the ball in the curve of your low back, with your tailbone untucked. Inhale to expand as you lower down, rolling with the ball and allowing your low back and bum to follow the curve of the ball so that your pelvis stays in neutral. Go down only as far as you feel comfortable (working up gradually to a full deep squat), and then exhale to engage and press back up to the starting point.

When you are ready to progress to a more challenging version of the exercise, take the ball away and repeat according to the photo below. Always inhaling as you lower down and exhaling as you press back up.

After you've had your baby, between weeks 4 and 6 postpartum, you can start doing the squats again, with the ball on the wall to start, keeping your range of motion small at first and gradually building back up to deeper squats.

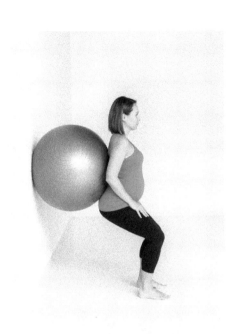

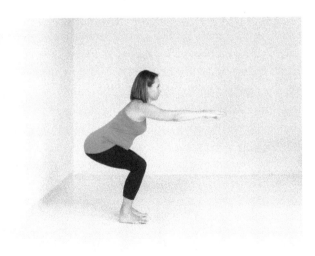

Shoulder Blade Retractions

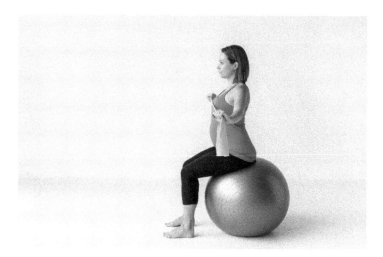

While not exactly training you for a specific birth position, this is an important exercise, especially for a soon-to-be-breastfeeding mom who will spend a lot of time during a typical day with very rounded shoulders. It is important to strengthen the upper back to help guide you to optimal posture.

Sit on your stability ball (or a chair, or you can even do this standing). Grasp a TheraBand, in the resistance level of your choice, with both hands about shoulder-width apart. Lift the arms and band up to shoulder height, keeping your arms straight. Inhale to expand, then exhale to engage and gently pull your hands away from one another so that the band stretches and moves closer to the chest while your arms are pulling the band straight out to the sides. Inhale to expand as you allow your arms to return to the start. Do 10–12 repetitions, 1–2 sets per day.

Postpartum, you can add this exercise in around week 3 or once you feel ready.

Seated One-Leg Lift

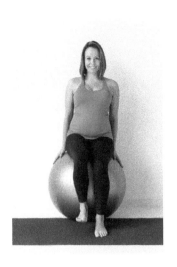

This is a great overall core exercise and helps build and maintain stability in the pelvis. Postpartum, it helps regain stability and prepares you for a return to more demanding exercises.

When you first start to do this exercise, wedge your ball into a corner or have it pressed up against a wall. Sit on your ball with your hands to the side for support. Inhale to expand, then exhale to engage and lift your right foot off the ground about 6 inches. Inhale and lower the leg back down. Do 10–12 repetitions and then repeat on the other side; 1–2 sets per day is ideal.

Postpartum, you will add this exercise in around week 5 or 6 or when your perineum feels ready.

Standing One-Leg Lift

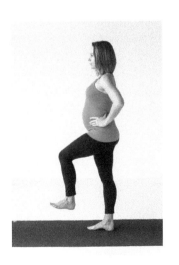

This exercise is a progression from the seated one-leg lift and is helpful in building core strength as well as strength and endurance in the legs for the standing labour positions. It is also a great exercise for pelvic stability.

Stand with your feet pelvis-width apart, with your hands on your hips and your pelvis in neutral. Inhale to expand, then exhale to engage and lift your left foot off the floor about 6 inches. Inhale and lower the leg back down. Try to keep the pelvis as neutral and stable as possible. Do 10–12 reps and then repeat on the other side, 1–2 sets per day.

If you notice that your pelvis "sinks" or drops to one side or wobbles, then don't lift your foot as high or simply go back to the seated version.

Note: If you have symphysis pubis dysfunction (SPD), please avoid this exercise.

Postpartum, you can add this exercise back in around week 5 or 6.

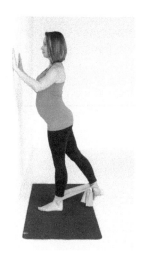

Hip Extensions

This simple but effective exercise helps build stability in the pelvis and also builds great glutes. Glutes are also great for the pelvic floor and will prevent the dreaded "mum bum"!

Tie a TheraBand in the resistance of your choice around your ankles. Stand facing a wall or hold onto a chair or stair banister for support. Shift your weight onto your left leg and lift your right foot slightly off the floor. Inhale to expand, then exhale to engage and press the right leg back, keeping the leg straight. Go as far as you can without leaning forward. Inhale and bring the leg back to the start.

Do 10–12 reps and then repeat on the other leg. Per day, 1–2 sets per leg is great!

Note: If you have symphysis pubis dysfunction (SPD), please avoid this exercise.

Postpartum, you can add this exercise in around six to eight weeks postpartum.

Stationary Lunge

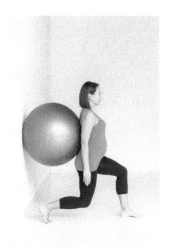

Lunging is one of those moves that is both very functional and a great overall exercise. You can do lunges with a ball for more stability, or you can hold onto a chair or a stair banister. You can also do them with no support at all, as in the second photo.

Lunging will help prepare you for the supported standing birth position and all of the picking up you will do in motherhood.

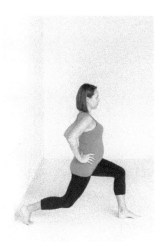

Take a nice wide split stance with one foot in front and the other behind. Inhale to expand as you lower down, then exhale to engage and press back up to the start. Do 10–12 reps per side, 1–2 sets per day.

Note: If you have symphysis pubis dysfunction (SPD), please avoid this exercise.

Postpartum, you can add this exercise back in around six to eight weeks.

***

Consider these birth preparation exercises as a moving meditation: take time for yourself to prepare your mind and body. The more you practise, the more the exercises will become normal and fluid, and the better prepared you will be for the big day!

Release for Birth

Let's look now at the stretch and release work that is as important as the exercises, if not more so.

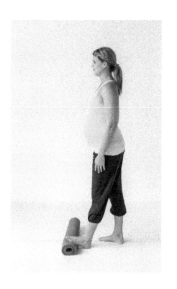

Calf Stretch

The calf and hamstring muscles are often tight because of all the sitting we do day to day as well as the shoes we wear. (I am a big supporter of minimalist shoes and ditching your heels is one of the best things you can do for your body!) Keeping length in the backside of the legs will help keep your pelvis optimally aligned, meaning better core function, better sacral position, and less SI joint pain.

Take a rolled-up towel or yoga mat and place it on the floor. Place the heel of your foot on the floor and the padded part of the foot at the base of the toes on the mat. Keep your body upright and the leg straight. Eventually, you should be able to step forward with the other foot (as if you were walking) while keeping the heel down, toes on the mat, and leg straight.

Hold for 30–60 seconds then repeat on the other side. Doing this several times throughout the day is best.

Postpartum, you can do this as soon as you wish.

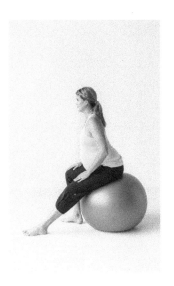

Hamstring Stretch

If you haven't already gathered, I like a stability ball. It has so many uses during pregnancy, is good to use in birth, and is a must-have for soothing your new baby with gentle bounces!

We just lengthened the calf, so now let's get a little higher up on the leg—the hamstrings. For all the same reasons mentioned earlier, this is an exercise you will want to do daily.

Sit on your stability ball with a neutral pelvis and an upright torso. Place your left leg out in front of you, and then hinge forward at your hip crease while pressing your bum backward on the ball. To increase the stretch, you can lift your toes up and place your heel on the floor. You can do this on a chair as well—ideally one that has a relatively hard surface, so you aren't sinking into a cushion. I like the ball because it allows you to really increase the length in the leg by pressing back on the ball as you hinge forward.

Hold for 30–60 seconds and then repeat on the other side. Do this several times a day.

Postpartum, you can do this as soon as your perineum feels up to it, and if you want to start right away, just sit at the edge of a chair to avoid pressure on the healing perineum.

Inner Thigh Stretch

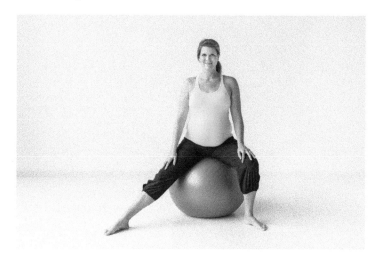

I talk a lot about keeping space in the pelvis during pregnancy and for birth. Stretching the inner thighs helps release tension and create space in the pelvis.

Sit on your stability ball with a neutral pelvis. If you are feeling unsteady, wedge the ball into a corner of the room. Keeping your left leg bent, extend your right leg straight out to the side and then press into your right foot so that you shift to your left on the ball. Feel amazing length created in the extended leg!

Hold for 30–60 seconds, and do several times daily.

Postpartum, you can return to this exercise once your perineum has healed and sitting on the ball is comfortable. You can always sit on the edge of a chair until the perineum is healed.

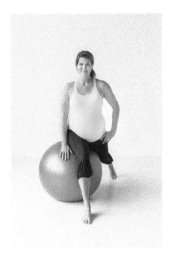

Hip Flexor Stretch

You and everyone you know should do this stretch several times a day. The front of the hips become very tight from the amount of sitting we do on a daily basis. Keeping the hip flexors (more specifically, the psoas muscle) long and tension free can optimize the position of the pelvis and the rib cage, leading to better fetal position, optimal breathing and core function, and less back pain.

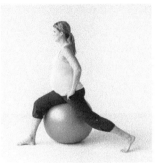

Side view of hip flexor stretch

Wedge the ball into a corner or press it up against a wall the first few times you do this. Sit on the side of the ball—meaning, take your right butt cheek and sit on the ball with the right knee bent and right foot on the floor in front. Extend your left leg back so that the leg is straight and the toes are on the floor. The first photo is the front view, and the second is the side view.

Keep the torso upright and think of increasing the space between your feet to generate length and release tension along the psoas muscle and the front of the hips.

Hold for 30–60 seconds, then repeat on the other side. Do this several times daily.

Postpartum, you can do stretch this once your perineum has healed.

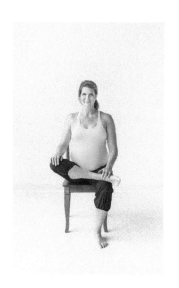

4-Stretch

Releasing tension in all parts of the pelvis and hips is key. Another typically tight part of the body is the side of the hips. The 4-stretch helps address this. Sit on a hard-surfaced chair with a neutral pelvis. Keeping the left foot planted on the floor, cross your right ankle over the left knee while trying to maintain your neutral pelvis. This alone may be enough of a stretch. If you want to increase the stretch, you can hinge forward at the hip.

Hold for 30–60 seconds then repeat on the other side. Do this several times daily.

Postpartum, you can do this stretch as soon as your perineum allows.

Seated Chest Opener

With all the driving and texting and computer using and dishwashing and cooking and so on that we do each day, the chest and front of the shoulders become very tight. Once you start breastfeeding, you will be adding another "in front of you" activity, so you'll want to keep the chest and shoulders loose and free!

Place a folded towel over the back of a hard (not cushioned)

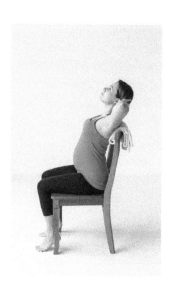

chair. Sit down and place your hands behind your head and your bum against the back of the chair. Slowly press your shoulder blades into the towel and look up at the ceiling, keeping your elbows wide. Feel the amazing expansion in the front of your chest and shoulders.

Hold for 30–60 seconds, several times daily.

Postpartum, you can initially do this lying down and then, when your perineum allows, seated.

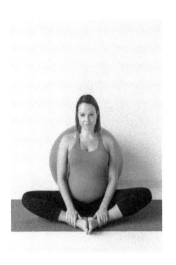

Butterfly

Not many people have the ability to do the butterfly without their tailbone tucked under them. I generally have people do this exercise seated, either against a wall or with the ball against the wall. The ball will help make sure you maintain the gentle curve in your low back. Sit with your back against the ball (or the wall) and bring your feet together in front of you. Keep your tailbone untucked and sit on your sitz bones—even if it means having your feet farther out in front of you. Now just sit and allow tension to release and openness to come. The muscles and tissues continue to lengthen and release as you do this. The key with release work is to *allow* rather than *do*. Release work should be done daily, even multiple times a day in a quiet spot where you can allow for 1–3 minutes each—Bliss!

Small Ball Release

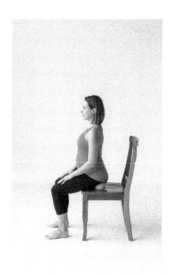

Another great way to open and lengthen during pregnancy is through the use of small balls. There are Franklin Balls, Miracle Balls, and Yoga Tune Up Therapy Balls. Franklin and Miracle balls are my faves to start with, as they have more squish and give to them, so using them is not quite as intense. Yoga Tune Up balls are a bit more dense and are actually my favourite to use for this exercise, but they may be better suited for use after you have done this exercise for a while with the softer balls.

Sit on a hard-surfaced chair or a bench. Lift up your left butt cheek and find your sitz bone, and put the ball in between your sitz bone and your anus. Now let your butt cheek settle back down. You may feel as though you are sitting unevenly—this is common. As you release, you will feel more balanced. Simply sit and think about allowing, and melting, and releasing. You're trying to keep space and suppleness in the pelvic floor, in that bowl of muscle in the pelvis.

Hold for 60–120 seconds. Really take the time to melt and release into the ball. Now take the ball out and notice the difference between the side you just released and the other side. Does your butt cheek feel wider, softer, flatter? Take note of the differences and then repeat on the other side.

Do this 2–3 times a day.

Postpartum, you will return to this once the perineum is fully healed.

Lying Side-Body Stretch

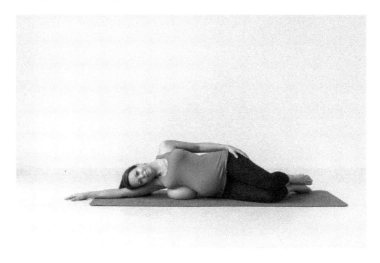

This next exercise will help you to create some length in your side body. The diaphragm is such an important part of the core and in breathing. In pregnancy, there is less space for your diaphragm because of the growing baby. You want to try to keep space and openness here so that you can breathe, and when you breathe better, your whole core works better.

For this exercise you will want to use a small ball that is half-inflated so that it has give. Lie down on your side and, if you want, take your bottom arm and put it underneath your head so you have a bit of support there. Roll back slightly, put the ball just underneath your ribs, and then roll forward onto the ball.

Think of allowing, lengthening, and melting over the ball. You can play around a little bit with the position of where that ball is; it might feel more tight in one spot than another. Remember to try and do this daily for 1–3 minutes per side.

Wide-Leg Child's Pose

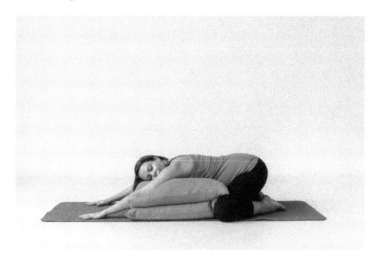

At the end of every day, I recommend you spend some time in the wide-leg child's pose—several times a day, if you like. Use a bolster or a stack of pillows under your belly as shown, so that your belly can rest on something and there will be less influence of gravity on the linea alba.

There is nothing to do in this pose but just be. Relax and let go.

If you had a hard time feeling and connecting to the core breath in sitting, the wide-leg child's pose can help. The openness of the pelvis and the stretched perineum can help facilitate feeling the movement of the breath with the pelvic floor.

***

So there you have it—exercises that will both prepare you for birth and help you restore form and function postpartum. Remember to start gradually. Honour the body. Don't feel like you need to do every single one of these exercises every single day. Start with one and see how you feel, then gradually add on as you feel ready.

In regards to cardio activity, here are a few of my favourites to help get your heart rate up while honouring the increasing weight of the growing baby.

Walking, especially hill walking, is one of the best exercises out there. It is a really good glute builder, and strong glute muscles will help keep your tailbone untucked.

When we live with the tailbone tucked, the glutes shut off. That's why you see a lot of new moms with flat pancake butts: when the tailbone is tucked, the glutes are inhibited, so they lose their bootiness.

Treadmill walking is a last resort—choose instead to get outside in nature and move your body naturally. Treadmills actually encourage the flat bum and glute inhibition because the tread is pulled back for us: instead of using our glutes to push off the ground to propel ourselves forward (like we are intended to do), we have to instead lift our foot and reach it forward as the other leg is being pulled back. This is not natural. Walking outside on uneven terrain and with some hills is the best thing you can do, pregnant or not.

If you can't get outside, the elliptical is the next best choice for cardio, as it is low impact and can get your heart rate up in a closer-to-natural way than the treadmill.

Swimming is a great low-impact activity that can feel heavenly in later pregnancy. The buoyancy of the water helps take weight off the joints, and the water can be a great place to explore hip-circling and leg-circling movements to maintain mobility in the pelvis.

So we have looked at safe and functional exercises that will help you prepare and recover from pregnancy and birth. We need to now look at exercises you should avoid.

Exercises to Avoid during Pregnancy

Crunches

Crunches shorten the front side of the body, which is not
something you need more of. Crunches also round the shoulders
and encourage a forward head position—again, not what you need
more of, especially given that you will be spending a lot of time in
a rounded shoulder, forward head position when you breastfeed.
Crunches also increase intra-abdominal pressure and strain the
linea alba (which in pregnancy is already strained enough!). They
can create a diastasis or make an existing one worse, so this is
definitely an exercise to avoid during pregnancy and once your
baby is born (and for the rest of your life, for that matter!).

Getting Up from a Back-Lying Position

Just like crunches are bad, so too is getting up from a lying-down
position by lifting your head and shoulders up and then pressing
into your hands to get up. Instead, roll to the side and then push
yourself up to seated. This goes for pregnancy and postpartum
(and once you've had a baby you are always postpartum... if you get
my drift).

The Plank

I generally caution pregnant women to stay away from positions
that are on all fours. The reason is that the growing baby and belly
are pushing against your connective tissue already. If you then
turn the belly down, you will add the pull of gravity, which will
add even more strain to the abdominals and connective tissue. I
do not recommend planks during pregnancy or in the early weeks
and months postpartum. Many people turn to planks if crunches
are off the table, but the plank is a really advanced exercise, and
if you are not strong enough to hold it and you have a weakened
linea alba and an abdominal separation, then your insides will
bulge or cone, which is not good. The plank is something that
you will work your way back to, but it's not your go-to exercise for

getting your abs back. Restore your core first and then gradually progress back to planks after the green light from your pelvic floor physiotherapist.

V-Sit

Avoid in pregnancy and after. This is an incredibly advanced exercise and, in my opinion, even after you have restored your core, it is not something I would have in your repertoire. It places a lot of strain on the back and abdomen and can increase intra-abdominal pressure, which is something you want to avoid during pregnancy and after.

Boat Pose

Just as the V-sit is not advised, neither is the boat pose. In fact, any exercise that has you lift both legs off the ground while you are either seated or lying should be avoided during pregnancy and after.

Pilates 100s (and other flexion movements)

While these are not a traditional crunch, they still involve the head being lifted off the ground and increase intra-abdominal pressure. If you have a diastasis, then there will be bulging at the belly and downward pressure on the pelvic floor. As such, this is another one to avoid both during and after pregnancy.

Jumping or Running

Running and jumping are activities that can place tremendous loads on the increasingly unstable pelvis. Your pelvic floor is working harder under the ever-increasing load of pregnancy. In my opinion it doesn't make sense to add high impact to this vulnerable area. Once the baby is born it is critical to allow time to heal (which can take months, even years by the way). I recommend avoiding high-impact activities for at least four to six months, and it is best to get cleared by your pelvic floor physiotherapist prior to reintroducing them into your routine.

Heavy Weight Lifting

Weight lifting is great for building muscle, but if the weight is too heavy, it can cause breath holding, which increases intra-abdominal pressure. Heavy weights can also lead to poor form as the body fatigues, which can wreak havoc on the healing core. Stick to lighter weights and do more repetitions. When you are doing weights, you can add in your core breath to many of the moves—for instance, a bicep curl. Inhale to expand with the weights in your hands at your sides, then exhale through pursed lips to engage the pelvic floor, then curl your hand weights up. For a chest press, inhale to expand to prepare, then exhale through pursed lips to engage the core and press the weights away from the chest. Pretty much any exercise you can do with the core breath means you are bringing your core into everything that you do!

Preparing the Foundation (Your Pelvic Floor) for Birth

We have incorporated the pelvic floor into the exercises by adding the core breath, but is that enough? Here are some other steps you can take to prepare your pelvic floor for birth.

Let's face it: a common thought that goes through the minds of many women is "How am I going to get something as big as a baby out of something as small as my vagina?"—followed by: "Will I be able to hold a tampon or my menstrual cup in?" "Will I still enjoy sex?" "Will pee fall out of me?" Women birthed babies long before there was prenatal education or hypnobirthing or this book, and, yes, the body is designed to give birth, but I believe it does take a little preparation, because an element of fear runs through the mind of every pregnant woman. I believe that a touch of fear is good because it can motivate and move you to take action, but when fear takes over, it can lead to problems. By preparing to push and empowering your mind and body, you are less likely to have fear ruling your birth and more likely to have the birth you want, without all the postpartum challenges like incontinence and diastasis.

I also believe we need some preparation because the lifestyle we lead now is much different from our grandmother's and her mother's. We move far less, we sit far more, and our posture and alignment take a beating. Because our posture and alignment are out of whack, our core is not working as it should. And when you then add on a pregnancy and birth, it can be a recipe for core function disaster. I believe that many "stalled" labours and "my pelvis was too small" scenarios and "the baby was not progressing" comments are actually a result of a dysfunctional core and poor birthing practices and perhaps fear. By maintaining ideal core function during pregnancy (ideally even before pregnancy), learning effective birth positions and breathing practices, and honouring the body as it heals postpartum, I believe that birth can take less of a toll on the modern-day body. So let's look a little more closely at how you can prepare your pelvic floor for birth.

Core Breath

The first tip we have already covered in detail—the core breath. By doing the core breath throughout your pregnancy, you will help maintain function and prevent dysfunction. Core breathing also enables you to connect with the movement of your pelvic floor. The exhale is the contraction and muscular activity portion of the breath, while the inhale is the relaxing and letting-go portion of the breath. This is key for giving birth: you need to know how to relax your pelvic floor, as this will enable you to keep space in the pelvis for your baby and also prevent your baby from meeting the resistance of a tight pelvic floor as it is trying to move through the birth canal.

Perineal Massage

Another tool to help you learn to relax, especially when you feel discomfort, is perineal massage. You can do this by yourself, or you can have your partner do it. (Both options are shown in the images here.)

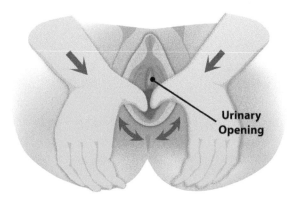

When performing perineal massage on your own, lubricate your thumbs with a natural oil such as olive or coconut. Lay in a semi-reclined position with your feet on the floor or bed and your knees bent. Reach down and place your thumbs at the entrance to the introitus (the vagina). Slowly and gently, press slightly down and then out and then up—almost like a U shape—and then hold with gentle pressure for several minutes. Release and repeat. Do this for over 10 minutes, and do it daily. Visualizations of softness and openness and fluidity will be helpful. Stay within your limits: this should not be painful—uncomfortable, yes, but not painful.

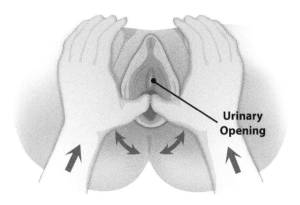

Urinary Opening

When your partner is performing perineal massage for you, he or she will sit or lie looking at your vulva, and use the same steps as above—lubricate, apply gentle pressure down, out, and then up in a U shape, and then hold it while you breathe softness into the space. This requires communication. Your partner will perhaps feel a bit hesitant at first, so talk through it and tell your partner "more" or "less" as needed.

Perineal massage, while beneficial, can be challenging to do on your own, and not every partner is willing to assist. Not only that, but there is no immediate feedback about progress to know if you have made any improvements.

The EPI-NO

My favourite way to train the pelvic floor and prepare the foundation is with the EPI-NO. It is much easier than perineal massage, gives immediate feedback and progress, and has been shown to be more effective than perineal massage.

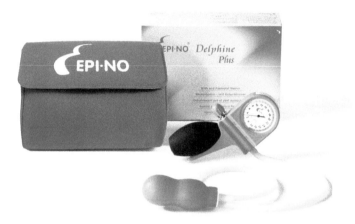

I used this personally in both of my pregnancies, and it is because of the EPI-NO that I am now doing what I do! It was my introduction to preventive and restorative pelvic health, and I will be forever grateful that I used and continue to use this amazing device. Yes, I sell these, but I can honestly say from experience that the EPI-NO is awesome, and here's why...

Studies have shown that EPI-NO users have a higher rate of intact perineum than non-users. The graph here shows some comparisons.

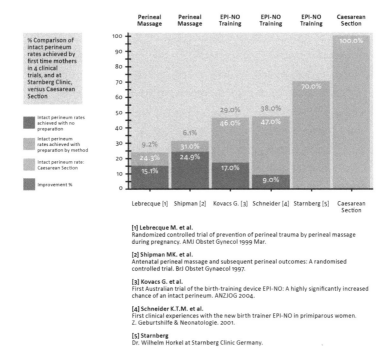

	Perineal Massage	Perineal Massage	EPI-NO Training	EPI-NO Training	EPI-NO Training	Caesarean Section

% Comparison of intact perineum rates achieved by first time mothers in 4 clinical trials, and at Starnberg Clinic, versus Caesarean Section

Intact perineum rates achieved with no preparation

Intact perineum rates achieved with preparation by method

Intact perineum rate: Caesarean Section

Improvement %

100.0%

70.0%

29.0%
46.0%

38.0%
47.0%

6.1%

9.2%
24.3%
15.1%

31.0%
24.9%

17.0%

9.0%

Lebrecque [1] Shipman [2] Kovacs G. [3] Schneider [4] Starnberg [5] Caesarean Section

[1] Lebrecque M. et al.
Randomized controlled trial of prevention of perineal trauma by perineal massage during pregnancy. AMJ Obstet Gynecol 1999 Mar.

[2] Shipman MK. et al.
Antenatal perineal massage and subsequent perineal outcomes: A randomised controlled trial. BrJ Obstet Gynaecol 1997.

[3] Kovacs G. et al.
First Australian trial of the birth-training device EPI-NO: A highly significantly increased chance of an intact perineum. ANZJOG 2004.

[4] Schneider K.T.M. et al.
First clinical experiences with the new birth trainer EPI-NO in primiparous women. Z. Geburtshilfe & Neonatologie. 2001.

[5] Starnberg
Dr. Wilhelm Horkel at Starnberg Clinic Germany.

1. The EPI-NO can shorten the pushing phase (second stage) of labour.

2. It is used during pregnancy to prevent and after pregnancy to restore.

3. The biofeedback aspect helps you connect with your ability to contract *and* your ability to relax.

4. It makes perineal massage much simpler to do; it involves the tissue around the entire vaginal opening, not just the bottom portion; and it has a measurement template, so you can see your progress!

The EPI-NO just makes sense to me... preparing for a physical event is a given in any other situation. If you think about running a marathon, for example, would you just wake up and go run the race? No, you would prepare. If you wanted to do a triathlon, you would train. If you wanted to climb Kilimanjaro, you would train.

Why then, for one of the most physically and mentally challenging events in a woman's life, is no thought given to preparing the body?

EPI-NO stands for "no episiotomy," and it was designed by a German physician who saw women in Africa using gourds of increasing size to prepare their perineum and pelvic floor for labour. He thought, "Cool, how do we make that more mainstream?" He worked with physiotherapists, doctors, and midwives and came up with the EPI-NO. It's a biofeedback silicon balloon. When it's deflated, it is about the size of a tampon. You lubricate yourself, the balloon, or both, and you insert it halfway into your vagina (there is an indentation to guide you). You close the nozzle and, with the black pump, you add a little bit of air. You add air until you feel like you have something to squeeze against. That's going to be at a different point for everybody, and it will be different for you on any given day depending on how much stress or tension you hold in your pelvic floor.

Once you have the balloon in place, you do your core breath or pelvic floor contractions. When you exhale and engage, you should see the needle on the gauge move. What you're looking for is that the needle goes up: Do you have the strength to make the needle go up? Do you have the endurance to hold it there for five seconds or so? And then do you have the ability to let go and allow the needle to come back down to where you started? It doesn't matter what number you are at when you put it in and inflated it. Whether it is at 6, or 12, or 2, it doesn't matter—it's just giving you a reference number as a starting point so you can monitor your ability to contract and then your ability to allow the needle to come back down to your starting point.

Do the EPI-NO biofeedback training every day for 10 minutes. In the last three weeks of pregnancy, add on 10 minutes of stretching and learn how to release and let go when you feel discomfort. This trains you for the point in actual birth when the baby's head is crowning. After you have done your 10 minutes of contracting and release work, leave the balloon inserted at the same point, and now inflate it to the point where you feel slight discomfort. It's not going to feel lovely, but it shouldn't hurt you. Hold it there for 10 minutes. The balloon is stretching the tissues around the entire vaginal opening. During that 10 minutes, you are breathing, you are visualizing, you are thinking about letting go and allowing. It does feel uncomfortable, but you need to learn how to yield to that discomfort. When it comes time to give birth to your baby, as the baby's head is crowning, there will be some discomfort, some tension, and you need to learn how to release and let go so that the baby has an easier time coming out and you are less likely to tear.

I liken the EPI-NO to Yin Yoga, which moves you into a pose and you are cued to "find your edge and stay there." You will find the point in the pose that feels pleasantly uncomfortable and then stay there allowing the tissues to release and let go. When you do the stretching phase with your EPI-NO, think of Yin Yoga—pump up the balloon until you "find your edge"—the pleasant discomfort —and stay there for 10 minutes allowing the tissues in the perineum to release and let go. At the end of the 10 minutes, relax the muscles enough so that the balloon can come out inflated. Again, it's giving you that sensation of allowing something to come out of you when you feel pressure and discomfort. Once it is out, measure the diameter of the balloon on the template that comes with it. The idea is that over the last three weeks, you should be able to inflate the balloon a little bit more each day, up to a 10-centimetre diameter, which is the same as the average circumference of a baby's head.

The first time I did the stretching, I was at 4.5 centimetres, and I got up to 9.5 centimetres before my first child was born. My son crowned sideways, which is the widest way a baby can crown. I didn't know it at the time, or it probably would have scared the heck out of me! But I had learned how to stay open and to yield, so I had no problems and I birthed through an intact perineum. My midwives told me afterward about his presentation, and they were amazed that I had no tearing and no abrasions. I credit them, because midwives definitely place a lot of attention on the perineum and on slowing things down. But I also place a lot of credit on the EPI-NO: it enabled me to have a mind–body connection, and I learned to allow things to let go even when I felt uncomfortable.

The EPI-NO is used restoratively after your baby is born, starting around six weeks. You do 10 minutes of the strengthening work to restore optimal function, and the key again is the balance of contracting and relaxing.

During pregnancy and during birth, there can sometimes be excessive stretch and pressure on the nerves. Most women have some element of nerve damage after they've had a vaginal or cesarean birth. When you have nerve damage, it affects the ability of the muscles to function as they should. It can also impair sensation, so postpartum, having the gauge on the EPI-NO can really help women reconnect to their pelvic floor—even if they don't feel anything, they can see what is happening.

A lot of women have a harder time relaxing, especially after they've had their baby. The EPI-NO is a great tool to help women learn how to relax just as much as it is a tool to help learn how to contract.

***

Women with placenta previa or vaginal varicosities or anybody who is not able to have sex during pregnancy should avoid both perineal massage and the EPI-NO. If you have a high-risk pregnancy, your doctor or midwife may caution you against this as well.

Visualization

Being able to connect with a part of your body that you can't see takes some visualization. Everyone is different, so what resonates with you will be completely different from what resonates with another woman. I generally use the following images to help women let go and release while doing perineal massage or during the stretching phase of the EPI-NO.

- Visualize a jellyfish softly floating in the water. Apply that image to your vagina and pelvic floor. Let go, soften and release tension, and float.

- Let go of any tension in the front of this hips, in the pelvis, in the groin, in the inner thighs, in the butt—let go and soften and release. Embrace the openness that you feel.

- Imagine that there is a drawstring that joins your pubic joint to your tailbone and to the sitz bones. Gradually loosen the cinch of the drawstring so that the bony points relax and move away from one another.

- Get a lava lamp and watch the globs in it melt and float. Allow that imagery to move to your abdomen and pelvis.

Remember when I told you that I would teach you a small modification to the core breath that you will practise in your last few weeks of pregnancy? Well, here it is... You will also take this with you into your labour and birth, so pay attention!

The core breath harnesses the true function of the core, in which the pelvic floor contracts with every exhale. During birth, however, you want to avoid consciously contracting the pelvic floor, because that would be like shutting the door on your baby. You need to keep the door open. So in the last few weeks of your pregnancy, you are going to modify the core breath slightly. You will still inhale to expand, creating space and openness in your pelvic floor, but as you exhale, you want to practise *keeping* that expansion in the pelvic floor. Your abdominals will still draw in (and should, because they are a key muscle for pushing), but your pelvic floor needs to stay free. It will be challenging at first, but keep at it.

Some element of contraction will happen naturally just because that's what the pelvic floor does, but you are taking out the voluntary contraction, and you want to try to imagine that that jellyfish is still nice and soft and open as you exhale.

If you have an EPI-NO, you can do this after you have done the stretching phase, paying attention to the gauge as you exhale and trying to have the needle move as little as possible. You can even practise a few gentle pushes once you have done a few breaths.

Once your baby is born, you will go back to the regular core breath to optimize the return to function.

CHAPTER SEVEN

Birthing Your Baby

Okay. We have looked at core function, how to proactively prepare it. We have looked at birth positions, exercises that prepare you for those birth positions, and how to prepare your pelvic floor for birth. Now let's look at what to do during the birth itself.

A Soothing Environment

The first step is to create a calm birthing environment. Whether at home or in a hospital, it is ideal to birth where *you* feel safest and where you have the best chance of having a calm space in which you can birth without interruption and without fear. When you feel afraid or are constantly interrupted, it can impede the progress of your labour.

Try to create an environment in which you have the ability to relax and let go. If you are in a very brightly lit room with doctors, nurses, friends, and family coming and going, and with many interruptions, how can you focus? Try to create an intimate space that is dimly lit, that is warm, and that has very little interruption. Some suggestions to think about relate to your senses:

- *Sound.* Do you want music or silence?

- *Taste.* Think of some snacks to have on hand for nourishment.

- *Smell.* Consider aromatherapy, and choose smells that you like, instead of choosing the ones that are recommended. Choose smells that bring you a sense of peace and calm.

- *Sight.* Harsh, bright lights can impede your labour, so opt instead for dimly lit spaces or rooms.

- *Touch.* Acupressure can be very helpful during labour, as can gentle massage or stroking. Warm compresses on the perineum may be soothing as your baby's head is crowning. Some women find that touch is distracting, though, and would rather be left alone, untouched—and that's all right, too.

Think of what you would like for your birth and remember, when you are actually in labour, this may all change, and that is okay. It is *your* birth: you are in control, you are in charge. Ask for what you want. You are a powerful mama!

Move

Movement in labour is key, especially in stage one. Once you reach stage 2 and are ready to push you will most likely move into one of the positions that you connected with during your preparation. Keep in mind though that if you practised a certain position and then, once in actual labour, you find that it is not as effective or comfortable as you had hoped, try something new! You have a good library of positions, and maybe your body, if you listen to the signals it sends, will take you into a position that we didn't cover in this book.

Breathe

As obvious as that sounds, it is not as easy as you think. The natural tendency when you feel pain is to hold your breath. This increases tension, reduces blood flow, and actually increases the sensations of discomfort. Midwives and doulas are amazing and will coach you through this.

Surrender

A word I love to use when empowering women for birth is *surrender*. Be confident knowing that you have prepared your body, that it is a natural amazing process, and that you *can* do this. Surrender to the experience and be amazed at what an incredible body you have!

Pushing

When you begin pushing, it can actually bring a huge sense of relief. Many women are actually surprised to find that the part they feared the most is actually the most rewarding and is easier to manage than the contractions leading up to it. Remember the modified core breath both in your labour and when you are ready to push. During the first stage of labour, inhale to expand as you feel a contraction, then exhale and maintain expansion in your pelvic floor, visualizing space and openness for your babe to move into. During the second stage of labour (when you push), inhale to expand as you feel a contraction, then exhale and maintain expansion in your pelvic floor while drawing the abdomen inward to help your contracting uterus. As you exhale, think of releasing tension in the pelvic floor (keeping your jellyfish floating softly).

Spontaneous vs. Directed Pushing

Pushing is not holding your breath and counting to 10 until you turn purple, but rather opening up your pelvis and allowing your body and your baby to do what is natural. Push when you feel the urge, and not when someone tells you to. Ideally, you are exhaling through the push while keeping that jellyfish nice and soft and open. You are trying to facilitate what the body is already doing on its own. If you have an epidural, you will not feel the urge to push and will need to be directed, but you can still use your breath and visualizations as you do so.

Tension Is Your Enemy

Ideally, when the baby is crowning, you want to yield against the discomfort instead of tensing up with fear and pain. When you are afraid or tense, your jaw is typically clenched, your psoas muscle is tight, and your pelvic floor is contracted. Mind–body birthing involves surrendering to the amazing process of birth and working with your body, not against it.

Don't Push as the Head Is Crowning

Ask your doctor or midwife to tell you when the baby's head is crowning, and then hold off on pushing. Instead, inhale to expand, and exhale thinking of relaxing and softening and opening the door for your baby. Resist the urge to push as this will allow for gentle expansion of the tissues in the perineum, making it less likely that you will tear.

Make Noise

When your jaw is clenched, so is your pelvic floor, and this is not at all achieving the state of relaxation that we want. Keep your jaw relaxed and mouth open. Try making *shhh*, *ssssss*, and *ahhhh* noises.

CHAPTER EIGHT

Healing Your New Mama Body

Congratulations—you're a mommy! Let the healing begin!
What is key to remember is that even if you have had no tearing or abrasions, you still need time to heal and to restore. Here are some great restorative healing practices.

Respect the Need to Heal

Respect your body and the healing process, and ask for and accept help. Hire a postpartum doula and have family around. Instead of a baby gift, ask that someone pay for the services of a doula or for home delivery of meals—anything that will help you to get through those initial weeks.

Ice, Heat, Water, and Rest

I recommend ice for the first 24 hours. You can make your own homemade ice pack using one part rubbing alcohol and two parts water in a resealable plastic bag (I always recommend double bagging). You can use also freeze maxi pads (ideally, a brand like NatraCare or a similar brand that doesn't have the harsh chemicals and that uses organic cotton, or reusable menstrual pads such as Lunapads). Soak them in water, freeze them, take them out, and put them into your underwear. Another option if using maxi pads is to first soak them in perineal healing herbs, and then freeze them. You can even fill up a condom and freeze that. Whatever you are using as an ice pack, make sure the ice is not directly against your skin: take one of the million little baby cloths you have from shower gifts and place that between your skin and the pack.

After the first 24 hours, you can switch to heat, in the form of sitz baths. Several times a day, soak in a bath full of Epsom salts with or without some healing herbs (you can find some at the Mama Goddess Birth Shop).

Every time you go to the washroom, wash your perineum afterward with a peri bottle (a little squirt bottle). You can also use water infused with the healing herbs for this. The perineum and vulva will feel too tender to wipe. Drink lots of water and eat fibre to keep your stools soft so you can avoid straining on the already tuckered-out tissues. Lie down as often as possible to relieve those tired tissues and avoid having to deal with the influence of gravity. Have someone bring your baby and your food to you. Lie down, stay warm, and relax.

Restore with the Core Breath

Start your core breath as soon as possible after giving birth. You can start within hours if you want to, but honour your body and do it when it feels right.

Belly Wrapping

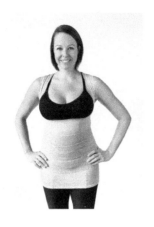

As I mentioned earlier, I strongly recommend wearing a support garment, which will help the connective tissue to heal. The one I recommend is the AB Tank, by Bellies Inc.; it provides support to the healing muscles and connective tissue as well as the low back and pelvis.

Mother Warming

A beautiful practice in many cultures—mother roasting, or mother warming—needs to be embraced in North America. Mother warming, based on the belief that women need to "close the body" after birth through rest and warmth, soothing massage, and belly wrapping, is such a nurturing and supporting custom but is unfortunately in stark contrast to the super-mom mentality in the Western world. Where mother warming is practised, trained practitioners often come to the home of a new mother to offer traditional ointments, baths, massages, and belly wrapping. Visit sacredpregnancy.com to find a certified mother roaster in your area.

Maya Abdominal Massage

Another wonderful restorative treatment is Maya Abdominal Therapy. This gentle, soothing massage can help the uterus settle back into the right position, improve circulation, and heal connective tissue. Visit arvigotherapy.com to learn more and to find a practitioner near you.

C-section Recovery

Caesarean births can be planned, which gives Mom time to prepare in advance for the procedure and for recovery. But in many cases, C-sections happen unexpectedly, leaving many women feeling surprised and overwhelmed. To make matters worse, little if any information is provided to new moms on how to recover properly.

C-section surgery involves cutting through the skin and underlying fat cells, the fascia (connective tissue), and the peritoneum (the lining of the abdominal cavity). The abdominal muscles are spread apart and an incision is made in the uterus to remove the baby. Once the baby is out, the incision in the uterus is sewn up, the fascia is sutured, and then, of course, the skin is stitched. That is a whole lot of layers of incisions and remaining scar tissue, not to mention some major alterations in the pelvic landscape!

If you are recovering from a Caesarean birth or know you will be having one, here are some tips on how to best recover and promote optimal healing:

- Supportive abdominal garments such as the AB Tank can be very beneficial and should be put on as soon as possible after the surgery. This will provide support to the incision, help the connective tissues heal, and encourage the abdominal muscles to realign.

- Rest and hydration are essential. Ask your family for help getting in and out of bed, walking to the washroom, getting on and off the toilet, and getting back into bed.

- Whenever you need to move, have someone assist you. Take a deep breath in. On the exhale, engage your core by contracting and lifting your pelvic floor, and then roll to your side. Take another breath in, exhale to engage your pelvic floor, and then use your arms to push yourself up while your assistant helps pull you up and move your legs over the side of the bed. Place your hands over your incision to support the area while you move. You should spend as little time as possible on your feet for the first few days—this will reduce the effect of gravity on the sutures, on the pelvic floor, and on the weak muscles and connective tissue. Don't rush. Take the time to heal.

- Do not lift anything heavier than your baby for the first few weeks. Heavy lifting and straining can damage weakened muscles and connective tissue while they are healing. Have family bring the baby to you for breastfeeding and cuddle time.

- Gentle point, flex, and circle movements of the foot and ankle can be done throughout the day while in bed to encourage blood flow, help reduce swelling, remove toxins, and minimize the risk of infection.

- Start gentle core breathing within the first few days to encourage maximum oxygen delivery to your recovering core. Inhale, allowing your ribs and belly to gently expand. Exhale gently through pursed lips to encourage the pelvic floor to engage. The exhalations will also help your body rid itself of any mucus that accumulated during the surgery. Proceed slowly and gently.

- Skin brushing encourages movement of fluids in the body, which can help reduce swelling. Using a soft bristle brush, gently stroke from your inner thigh up toward your heart. This can begin about two days postpartum and can be done several times daily.

- Scar tissue mobilization is important to prevent adhesions from building up in all of those layers of incision points. Adhesions can lead to decreased mobility and impaired core function. Mobilizing the scar will be done in the later weeks after the incision has healed. See a pelvic floor physiotherapist for initial assistance, and then practise daily at home. A great tool for releasing adhesions and promoting better function is the Coregeous Ball from Yoga Tune Up—its tacky surface grips the skin and can help mobilize stuck tissue.

- The six-week mark has generally been the golden "return to activity" date, but really there is no set date. Everyone heals differently. By six weeks you should be able to walk more freely, but vigorous activity, heavy lifting, and high-impact movements are still off limits. The focus remains on core restoration—because if the foundation is not restored, you will prevent proper healing of diastasis recti and increase the likelihood of suffering from incontinence and organ prolapse.

- Crunches are off limits! They encourage a pooch, they create pressure on the pelvic floor, and they promote a C-shaped posture, which is the last thing a breastfeeding mom needs!

- One last thing: *mommy* and *boot camp* do not belong in the same sentence (or other forms of vigorous exercise for that matter.)

Honour Your Body as It Heals

The postpartum period can be a frustrating time for women. Many of them want to jump right back into their former shape as soon as possible. They are joining boot camps and CrossFit. They are thinking it is a good time to run a marathon. They haven't even given their body time to heal, and with the core not working properly, they are adding loads onto weak, weak muscles. The best advice: take time to heal gradually. You *can* achieve the post-partum body you want, just not overnight.

CHAPTER NINE

Restorative Exercise for New Moms

FRONTAL SECTION OF PELVIS

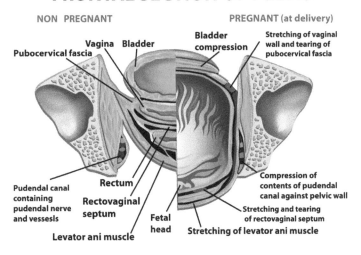

NON PREGNANT   PREGNANT (at delivery)

Pubocervical fascia — Vagina Bladder

Bladder compression — Stretching of vaginal wall and tearing of pubocervical fascia

Pudendal canal containing pudendal nerve and vessesls — Rectum

Rectovaginal septum

Fetal head

Compression of contents of pudendal canal against pelvic wall

Stretching and tearing of rectovaginal septum

Levator ani muscle   Stretching of levator ani muscle

For those of you who will have a vaginal birth, consider this photo and allow the image to influence your healing and eventual return to exercise. It is not realistic to think that at 6 weeks postpartum you are ready to return to 'normal' activities. Respect the magnitude of what your amazing body has done and appreciate that at 6 weeks, the healing has only just begun.

For the first two weeks, I recommend staying at home: breastfeed your baby, have lots of baths, lie down, and have other people take care of you and bring your baby to you. Feed yourself. Just take it easy. There's no rush.

Around two or three weeks postpartum, you can start slowly introducing some walking. Go back to the walking routes you were taking before, but start with just 10 or 15 minutes—ideally on a flat surface—and gradually increase from there.

Practise your core breathing for a concentrated 30 seconds to a minute each day.

Allow your core time to return to its optimal functioning. I recommend staying away from high-impact activities, including running, for at least four to six months. See a pelvic floor physiotherapist after six weeks. (Ideally, you should meet with a physiotherapist during your pregnancy as well.)

It is not realistic to think that at six weeks you are ready to jump or run or put your body through anything strenuous. Remember how long it took for your body to change during pregnancy? Remember that you also then gave birth? Your body has been through a lot, and regardless of how badly you want to get back to your regular routine and your old clothes, your body is simply not ready. Your body is injured, your core is compromised, and you need time to heal. Build yourself back up gradually.

I recommend just core breathing in your first week and then gradually add on. Use the postpartum protocol (coming up), but remember it is a guide, not a strict plan. Listen to your body and take it slow. You will gradually progress through the weeks, but if it ever feels like too much, just back up.

Restorative Exercise

Your postpartum recovery exercises are nearly the same as the ones you did while you were pregnant, only now you have your little bundle on the outside!

If you remember all the talk about alignment... well, not only is it just as important, it can be harder to maintain as you carry your babe. You want to aim for your pelvis over your ribcage. Keep your tailbone untucked and aim for the weight of your body to be in the midfoot, closer to the heal as opposed to forward in the toes.

Alignment comes first, then breathing (think core breath) and then coordination (think movement).

In the Prepare To Push™ e-course available at pelviennewellness.com you will find videos to help fine tune your alignment and movement.

Before we get to the Restorative Exercises I would like to discuss briefly an exercise method that I have come to love and highly recommend be done in conjunction with the exercises I outline in this book. The method is called Hypopressives, or Low Pressure Fitness. I first became aware of this technique through Kaisa Tuominen of postnatalbodyfix.com and tried to bring her to Canada. A year went by and we were no closer to finding a date. Then, a friend of mine who I had introduced to the world of pelvic floor health and fitness had recently found out she had a grade 2 bladder prolapse and was devastated. I told her to look up hypopressives which she did and started trying to teach herself the method from what was available online (which was limited at the time). She decided to travel to Spain to learn directly from Kaisa. Upon returning and practicing the protocol diligently, her prolapse went to a grade 1 and not long after it was gone. She was a believer and is now manager of Low Pressure Fitness in Canada. I became certified in level 1 and have used it with clients and myself with great success. You can learn more by visiting lowpressurefitness.com and hypopressivescanada.com.

Hypopressive Exercise

The HYPOPRESSIVE™ techniques were created in Europe in the early 1980s with the goal of helping postpartum women prevent and recover from pelvic floor dysfunctions such as incontinence and prolapse. The term 'HYPOpressive' refers to a decrease or reduction in pressure. This form of exercise, now being referred to as low pressure fitness, reduces pressure to the thoracic, abdominal and pelvic cavities, where traditional abdominal exercises, gravity, as well as the majority of our daily activities are HYPERpressive—they increase intra-abdominal pressure. We need some intra-abdominal pressured to help stabilize our spine but pregnancy and birth can interfere with our ability to manage these pressures and this is what can then lead to dysfunctions of the pelvic floor.

Hypopressives are a specific set of poses that create a decrease in pressure and amplify the hypopressive effects, lift the internal organs and improve posture. In the pose, an apnea (a temporary cessation of breathing) and then a false inhlale are added after a full exhale to create a vacuum affect resulting in a decrease of pressure within the thoracic, abdominal and pelvic cavities. The diaphragm acts like a plunger and the activation of its antagonist muscle, the serratus anterior, and the inspiratory muscles during the apnea and false inhale, causes a suction effect in as the diaphragm elevates. This decreases pressure and initiates an elevation of the tissues. It is an odd looking regime but very effective. It is best learned from a trainer as there are many points to perfect but once you learn it, you can practice daily on your own. As a final note, it is much more rigorous than it appears and is much more than a breathing technique. It is a challenging full body technique that is making headlines in the pelvic floor world. Check the resources section for links.

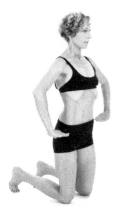

Image used with permission:
Trista Zinn HYPOPRESSIVES Canada

Posture Pointers

Classic New Mama Posture (not ideal)

- Hips thrust forward
- Tailbone tucked
- Glutes gripping
- Rib cage behind pelvis

Optimal New Mama Posture

- Hips over ankles
- Rib cage over pelvis
- Tailbone untucked

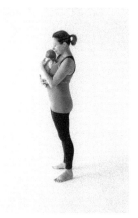 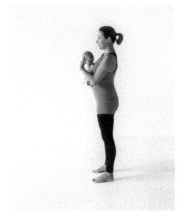

Same thing goes when you use your carrier:

Typical Posture with a Carrier

Optimal Posture with a Carrier

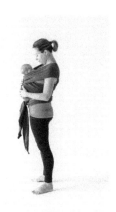 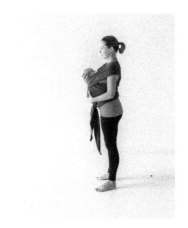

Your Postpartum Exercises

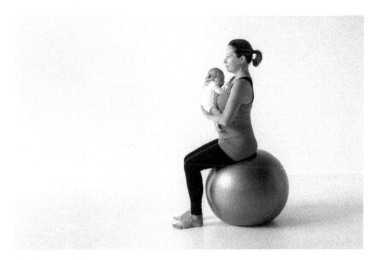

The Core Breath

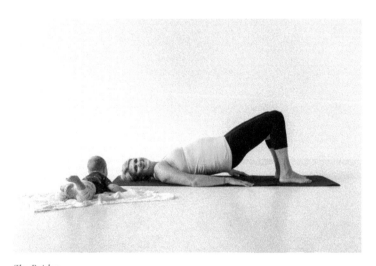

The Bridge

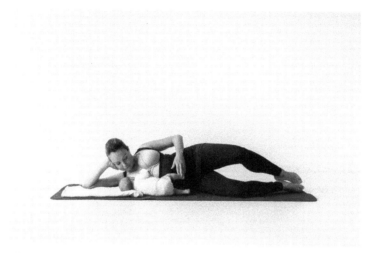

The Clam

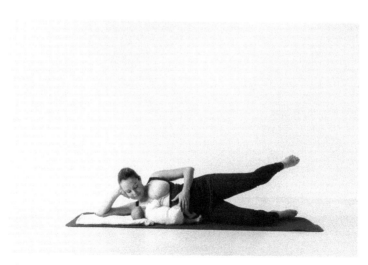

The Broken Clam

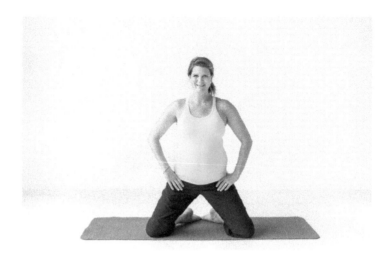

The Wide Kneel

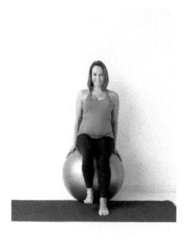

Seated One-Leg Lift

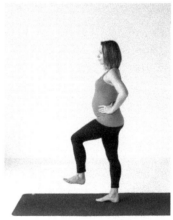

Standing One-Leg Lift

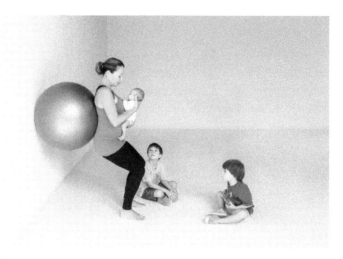

The Squat

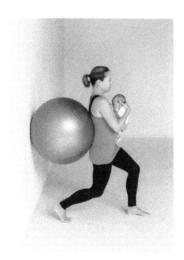

The Lunge

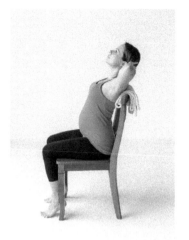

Seated Chest Stretch

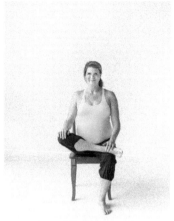

4-Stretch

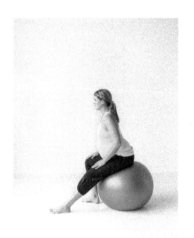

Hamstring Stretch

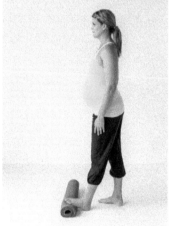

Calf Stretch

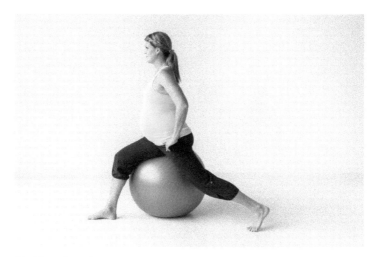

Hip Flexor Stretch

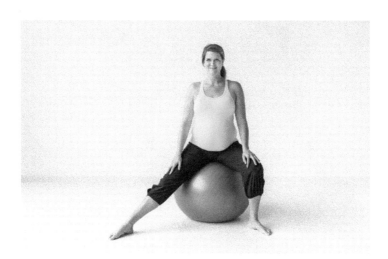

Inner Thigh Stretch

Postpartum Exercise, Week by Week

Week 1

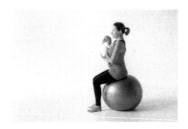

1. The Core Breath

Week 2

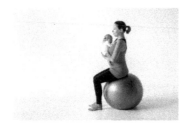

1. The Core Breath

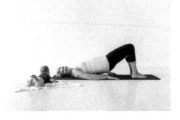

2. The Bridge

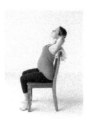

3. Seated Chest Stretch

Week 3

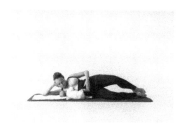

1. The Core Breath

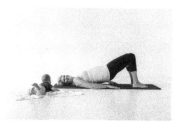

2. The Bridge

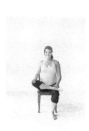

3. The Clam

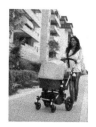

4. Seated Chest Stretch

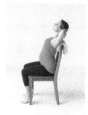

5. 4-Stretch

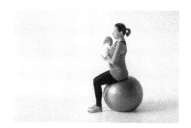

6. Gentle walk up to 20 minutes

Make an appointment to see your pelvic floor physio at six weeks. In fact, put the book down, and go pick up the phone and make the appointment right now, so you can take it off the list! Even if you are still pregnant as you read this, make the appointment now. Your health is important. *You* are important. Make *you* a priority.

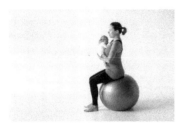

1. The Core Breath

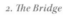

2. The Bridge

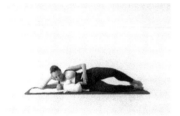

3. The Clam

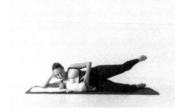

4. The Broken Clam

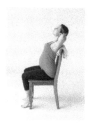

5. Seated Chest Stretch

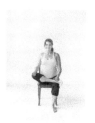

6. 4-Stretch

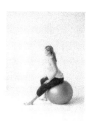

7. Hamstring Stretch

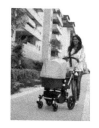

8. Gentle walk up to 20 minutes

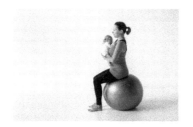

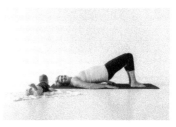

1. *The Core Breath*

2. *The Bridge*

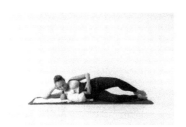

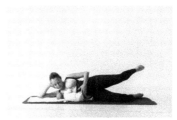

3. *The Clam*

4. *The Broken Clam*

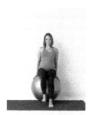

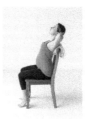

5. *Seated One-Leg Lift*

6. *Seated Chest Stretch*

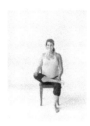

7. 4-Stretch

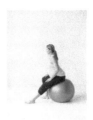

8. Hamstring Stretch

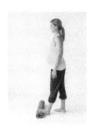

9. Calf Stretch

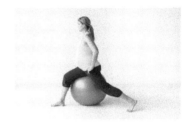

10. Hip Flexor Stretch

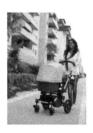

11. Gentle walk up to 20 minutes

See your pelvic floor physio.

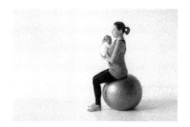

1. The Core Breath

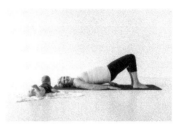

2. The Bridge

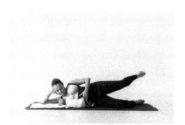

3. The Broken Clam

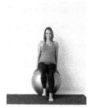

4. Seated One-Leg Lift

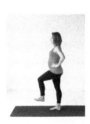

5. Standing One-Leg Lift

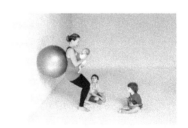

6. Squat

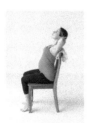

7. Seated Chest Stretch

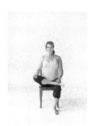

8. 4-Stretch

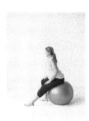

9. Hamstring Stretch

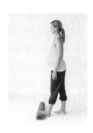

10. Calf Stretch

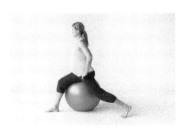

11. Hip Flexor Stretch

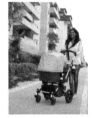

12. Moderate walk up to 30 mintues

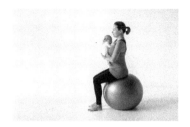

1. *The Core Breath*

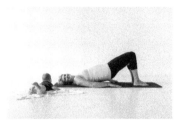

2. *The Bridge*

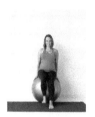

3. *Seated One-Leg Lift*

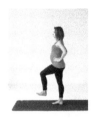

4. *Standing One-Leg Lift*

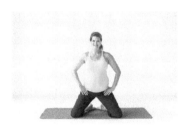

5. *Wide Kneel*

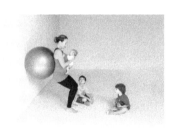

6. *Squat*

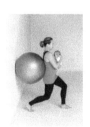

7. *The Lunge*

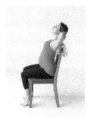

8. *Seated Chest Stretch*

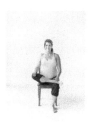

9. 4-Stretch

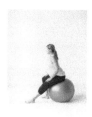

10. Hamstring Stretch

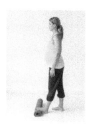

11. Calf Stretch

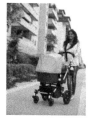

12. Hip Flexor Stretch

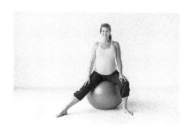

13. Inner Thigh Stretch

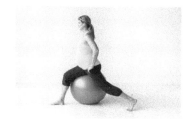

14. Moderate walk up to 40 mintues

You are on an incredible journey into motherhood and having taken the time to read through this book you are now armed with information that will foster a better birth and recovery. Embrace the journey and feel confident knowing that you are honouring your body through this amazing process.

Prepare To Push™ is also available as an eCourse at preparetopush.com. The content is expanded upon and videos help foster deeper learning.

So there you have it—consider yourself prepared to push! May you find strength and comfort in your pregnancy, joy in your birth and confidence in motherhood.

Resources

AB Tank
belliesinc.com

Babybellyband
babybellyband.com

Baby Belly Belt
babybellybelt.com/about-diane-lee.php

EPI-NO
pelviennewellness.com/collections/pregnancy/products/epi-no-delphine-plus

EPI-NO International
epi-no.com

Franklin Method
franklinmethod.com/products1/equipments

The Hypopressive Method
hypopressivescanada.com/
lowpressurefitness.com/

Miracle Balls
elainepetrone.com

Mama Goddess Birth Shop
mamagoddessbirthshop.com

MuTu
mutusystem.com

TheraBand
thera-band.com/store/index.php

Yamuna
yamunausa.com

Yoga Tune Up
yogatuneup.com

Find a Pelvic Floor Physio

Canada
pelviennewellness.com/apps/find-physio

USA
Choose Women's Health
apta.org/apta/findapt/index.aspx?navID=10737422525

Find a Doula

Canada
cappa.net/canada.php

USA
cappa.net

Find a Midwife

Canada
cmrc-ccosf.ca/node/21

USA
midwife.org/find-a-midwife

References

Balaskas, Janet. (1992). *Active Birth*. Boston: Harvard Common Press.

Bowman, Katy. (2013). *Alignment Matters: The First Five Years of Katy Says*. Ventura, CA: Propriometrics Press.

Calais-Germain, Blandine, and Nuria Vives Pares. (2009). *Preparing for a Gentle Birth: The Pelvis in Pregnancy*. Rochester, VT: Healing Arts Press.

Goldberg, Roger. (2003). *Ever Since I Had My Baby*. New York: Three Rivers Press.

Koch, Liz. (2012). *The Psoas Book*. Felton, CA: Guinea Pig Publications.

Lynn, Valerie. (2012). *The Mommy Plan*. Kuala Lumpur, Malaysia: Percetakan Lenang Istimewa Sdn Bhd.

Murphy, Magnus, and Carol L. Wasson. (2003). *Pelvic Health & Childbirth*. Amherst, NY: Prometheus Books.

Palm, Sherrie J. (2009). *Pelvic Organ Prolapse: The Silent Epidemic*. New York: Eloquent Books.

CPSIA information can be obtained
at www.ICGtesting.com
Printed in the USA
LVHW02s2336180218
566944LV00007B/7/P